Psychiatric Nursing:
Current Trends in Diagnosis and Treatment

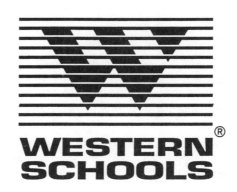

WESTERN
SCHOOLS®

By
Bethany A. Murray, APRN, BC

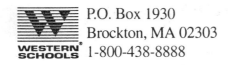
P.O. Box 1930
Brockton, MA 02303
1-800-438-8888

ABOUT THE AUTHOR

Bethany A. Murray is a practicing Advanced Practice Registered Nurse with her master's degree in child/adolescent, psychiatric and mental health nursing. She is credentialed by the American Nurse Credentialing Center as a Child Clinical Nurse Specialist. Ms. Murray has worked in the psychiatric field since 1986. She is currently the nursing manager at the Center for Behavioral Health in Bloomington, IN, as well as a part-time lecturer for the Indiana University School of Nursing. Ms. Murray is a member of the Coalition of Advanced Practice Nurses of Indiana (CAPNI), an educational and political organization that promotes advanced nursing practice at a local, state, and national level.

ABOUT THE SUBJECT MATTER REVIEWER

Lynette Jack is currently an associate professor in the School of Nursing at the University of Pittsburgh and director of Student Services for RN Options and Graduate Programs. Lynette received her master's degree in Psychiatric/Mental Health Nursing from the University of Pittsburgh in 1978 and her PhD in Higher Education, also from the University of Pittsburgh, in 1985. Lynette has taught Psychiatric Nursing to undergraduate students for 20 years and also teaches a graduate level course on the prevention and treatment of addictions. Lynette is currently president of the International Society of Psychiatric-Mental Health Nurses (ISPN).

Copy Editor: Julie Munden

Indexer: Sylvia Coates

ISBN: 1-57801-100-0

IMPORTANT: Read these instructions *BEFORE* proceeding!

Enclosed with your course book, you will find the FasTrax® answer sheet. Use this form to answer all the final exam questions that appear in this course book. If you are completing more than one course, be sure to write your answers on the appropriate answer sheet. Full instructions and complete grading details are printed on the FasTrax instruction sheet, also enclosed with your order. Please review them before starting. *If you are mailing your answer sheet(s) to Western Schools, we recommend you make a copy as a backup.*

ABOUT THIS COURSE

A Pretest is provided with each course to test your current knowledge base regarding the subject matter contained within this course. Your Final Exam is a multiple choice examination. **You will find the exam questions at the end of each chapter.**

In the event the course has less than 100 questions, mark your answers to the questions in the course book and leave the remaining answer boxes on the FasTrax answer sheet blank. Use a <u>black</u> **pen to fill in your answer sheet.**

A PASSING SCORE

You must score 70% or better in order to pass this course and receive your Certificate of Completion. Should you fail to achieve the required score, we will send you an additional FasTrax answer sheet so that you may make a second attempt to pass the course. Western Schools will allow you three chances to pass the same course...*at no extra charge!* After three failed attempts to pass the same course, your file will be closed.

RECORDING YOUR HOURS

Please monitor the time it takes to complete this course using the handy log sheet on the other side of this page. See below for transferring study hours to the course evaluation.

COURSE EVALUATIONS

In this course book, you will find a short evaluation about the course you are soon to complete. This information is vital to providing Western Schools with feedback on this course. The course evaluation answer section is in the lower right hand corner of the FasTrax answer sheet marked "Evaluation," with answers marked 1–19. Your answers are important to us; please take a few minutes to complete the evaluation.

On the back of the FasTrax instruction sheet, there is additional space to make any comments about the course, the school, and suggested new curriculum. Please mail the FasTrax instruction sheet, with your comments, back to Western Schools in the envelope provided with your course order.

TRANSFERRING STUDY TIME

Upon completion of the course, transfer the total study time from your log sheet to question 19 in the course evaluation. The answers will be in ranges; please choose the proper hour range that best represents your study time. You **MUST** log your study time under question 19 on the course evaluation.

EXTENSIONS

You have two (2) years from the date of enrollment to complete this course. A six (6) month extension may be purchased. If after 30 months from the original enrollment date you do not complete the course, *your file will be closed and no certificate can be issued.*

CHANGE OF ADDRESS?

In the event you have moved during the completion of this course, please call our student services department at 1-800-618-1670, and we will update your file.

A GUARANTEE TO WHICH YOU'LL GIVE HIGH HONORS

If any continuing education course fails to meet your expectations or if you are not satisfied in any manner, for any reason, you may return it for an exchange or a refund (less shipping and handling) within 30 days. Software, video, and audio courses must be returned unopened.

Thank you for enrolling at Western Schools!

WESTERN SCHOOLS
P.O. Box 1930
Brockton, MA 02303
(800) 438-8888
www.westernschools.com

Psychiatric Nursing: Current Trends in Diagnosis and Treatment

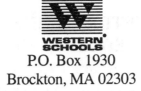

WESTERN SCHOOLS
P.O. Box 1930
Brockton, MA 02303

Please use this log to total the number of hours you spend reading the text and taking the final examination (use 50-min hours).

Date	Hours Spent
_____	_____
_____	_____
_____	_____
_____	_____
_____	_____
_____	_____
_____	_____
_____	_____
_____	_____
_____	_____
_____	_____
_____	_____
_____	_____

TOTAL [   ]

Please log your study hours with submission of your final exam. To log your study time, fill in the appropriate response under question 19 of the FasTrax® answer sheet under the "Evaluation" that follows.

Psychiatric Nursing: Current Trends in Diagnosis and Treatment

WESTERN SCHOOLS
CONTINUING EDUCATION EVALUATION

Instructions: Mark your answers to the following questions with a black pen on the "Evaluation" section of your FasTrax® answer sheet provided with this course. You should not return this sheet. Please use the scale below to rate the following statements:

A Agree Strongly   C Disagree Somewhat
B Agree Somewhat   D Disagree Strongly

The course content met the following education objectives:

1. Explained the epidemiology and history of mental health care and the diagnosing of psychiatric disorders.

2. Discussed some of the legal, ethical, and cultural issues associated with mental health care and treatment.

3. Explained a nursing history of a psychiatric patient and how to write an effective nursing care plan.

4. Identified symptoms of a thought disorder and discussed appropriate nursing care and medication treatment.

5. Identified the symptoms of a dementia disorder, differentiated it from delirium, and identified appropriate nursing measures for promoting safety and maximizing functioning.

6. Discussed alcoholism, sedative, hypnotic, and anxiolytic dependence in American society including the recognition and treatment of withdrawal syndromes.

7. Discussed drug dependency in American society including the recognition and treatment of withdrawal syndromes.

8. Identified symptoms of a depressive disorder and discussed relevant treatment including therapy and medications.

9. Identified symptoms of bipolar spectrum disorders and discussed appropriate nursing care and medication treatment.

10. Identified symptoms of an anxiety disorder and discussed relevant treatment including therapy and medications.

11. Recognized mental health disorders that are expressed by poor nutrition, medical complaints, or sleep problems.

12. Discussed problems associated with domestic violence and how they relate to the development of dissociative and personality disorders.

13. Discussed normal childhood development and recognized cognitive and emotional disorders that arise from disruptions in development.

14. Described disruptive behavior disorders and Tourette's disorder, and discussed relevant treatments.

15. The content of this course was relevant to the objectives.

16. This offering met my professional education needs.

17. The objectives met the overall purpose and goal of the course.

18. The course was generally well-written and the subject matter explained thoroughly. (If no, please explain on the back of the FasTrax instruction sheet.)

19. **PLEASE LOG YOUR STUDY HOURS WITH SUBMISSION OF YOUR FINAL EXAM.**
Please choose which best represents the total study hours it took to complete this 30-hour course.

A. Less than 25 hours

B. 25–28 hours

C. 29–32 hours

D. Greater than 32 hours

CONTENTS

FIGURES AND TABLES

Chapter 13

Chapter 14

PRETEST

1. Begin this course by taking the pretest. Circle the answers to the questions on this page, or write the answers on a separate sheet of paper. Do not log answers to the pretest questions on the FasTrax test sheet included with the course.

2. Compare your answers to the PRETEST KEY located in the back of the book. The pretest key indicates the course chapter where the content of that question is discussed. Make note of the questions you missed, so that you can focus on those areas as you complete the course.

3. Complete the course by reading each chapter and completing the exam questions at the end of each chapter. Answers to these exam questions should be logged on the FasTrax test sheet included with the course.

1. Of every 100 persons in the United States, the number diagnosed with schizophrenia is

   a. 5.

   b. 1.

   c. 30.

   d. 50.

2. Ethical principles are meant to

   a. guide the health care professional in decision-making.

   b. serve as rules for conduct in society.

   c. prevent errors in judgment.

   d. predict the behaviors of individuals.

3. The 14th Amendment guarantees the right to

   a. bear arms.

   b. vote.

   c. free speech.

   d. life, liberty, and property.

4. Data suggests that the overall rates of psychiatric disorders in minority populations in the United States are

   a. lower than in the general population.

   b. the same as the general population.

   c. higher than in the general population.

   d. not addressed in this study.

5. The four components of the nursing process are

   a. Assessment, Intervention, Education, Supervision.

   b. Assessment & Diagnosis, Care Planning, Intervention, Evaluation.

   c. Diagnosing, Planning Care, Evaluating Outcomes, Passing Medications.

   d. Treatment Planning, Taking off Orders, Giving Medications, Charting.

6. Schizophrenia is caused by

   a. neurobiological alterations yet to be identified.

   b. impoverished home environments.

   c. mentally ill mothers with domineering personalities.

   d. chronic drug and alcohol abuse.

7. The percentage of individuals over age 65 with a dementia disorder is

    a. 10-15%.
    b. 4-5%.
    c. 2-4%.
    d. 1%.

8. The chemical that causes the "hangover effect" of alcohol intoxication is

    a. acetaldehyde.
    b. ethanol.
    c. acetic acid.
    d. carbon dioxide.

9. Symptom sets associated with opioid withdrawal include

    a. hallucinations, paranoid delusions.
    b. neuron excitability, grand mal seizures.
    c. violent outbursts, followed by stupor.
    d. lacrimation, piloerection, muscle aches, rhinorrhea.

10. Prevalence rates for major depression in women are

    a. 1%.
    b. 5%.
    c. 10%.
    d. 40%.

11. *DSM-IV-TR* criteria for diagnosing major depression must include

    a. a depressed mood or a loss of interest or pleasure in activities.
    b. weight increases or decreases.
    c. suicidal thoughts or behaviors.
    d. irritability or grouchiness.

12. Symptoms of mania associated with a bipolar I disorder must include

    a. delusions and hallucinations.
    b. an abnormal and elevated, expansive or irritable mood.
    c. spending sprees and promiscuity.
    d. poor judgment, insight, or awareness of symptoms.

13. Diagnosing bipolar II disorder may take as long as

    a. 2 years.
    b. 5 years.
    c. 8 years.
    d. 12 years.

14. Generalized anxiety disorder is characterized by

    a. excessive worry about a variety of events or activities.
    b. specific fears of certain situations.
    c. hypervigilance and flashbacks.
    d. repetitive thoughts and actions.

15. Eating disorders often onset in

    a. early childhood.
    b. middle to late adolescence.
    c. college years.
    d. adulthood.

16. Narcolepsy is associated with

    a. excessive amphetamine abuse.
    b. problems with primary insomnia.
    c. a disturbance in REM sleep architecture.
    d. sleep apnea concerns.

17. Of women who are killed annually in the
    United States, the percentage that is secondary
    to domestic violence is

    a. 1-3%.

    b. 5-10%.

    c. 10-20%.

    d. 30-50%.

18. Erikson's 8 stages of growth and development
    include

    a. oral stage.

    b. trust versus mistrust.

    c. concrete operational thought.

    d. the Oedipal phase.

19. Attention-Deficit/Hyperactivity Disorder
    occurs in males at a rate that is

    a. 3-4 times higher than in females.

    b. twice as high as in females.

    c. the same as in females.

    d. half as much as in females.

20. The prevalence of Tourette's disorder is

    a. 1 in 1,000 children.

    b. 1 in 10,000 children.

    c. 4 in 1,000 children.

    d. 4 in 10,000 children.

INTRODUCTION

In the 1948 book *Psychiatry in Nursing* (Headlee & Corey) the psychiatric nurse is described as requiring an "entirely different set of values, new ways of thinking, new attitudes, and new techniques." The authors go on to say "making satisfactory contacts with human beings constitutes psychiatric nursing." Little has changed in the past 50 years regarding this basic humanistic approach. However, what has changed dramatically has been the nurse's ability to practice with increasing autonomy in providing care for clients, and to be perceived as an important member of the multidisciplinary health care team.

One of the purposes of this educational offering is to teach nurses about psychiatric disorders, various treatment modalities, therapeutic communication skills, medications, and cultural variances in the way mental illness is perceived and treated in both adults and children.

Psychiatric nursing utilizes a continuum of care model. Psychiatric clients are no longer found exclusively within the hospital setting. Every year, new medications are launched with improved efficacy and fewer side effects. Acute psychiatric hospital stays are becoming shorter, with many hospital stays lasting only 3-5 days (historically, clients were hospitalized for the duration of their illness — often up to 3 months in an acute care hospital before transferring to a long-term care facility). The separation of mental health care from medical/surgical care has become an artificial distinction. Nurses who believe that they will have no need for ongoing education in psychiatric disorders or their treatment may find themselves to be at a distinct disadvantage, as individuals with psychiatric diagnoses are encountered in all treatment areas.

It is the goal of this book to assist nurses in updating their mental health skills and knowledge of current psychiatric treatments. Nurses must recognize and be able to care for clients in inpatient, residential, outpatient or home settings, as well as numerous medical settings, such as nursing homes and primary practice offices. The concept of "least restrictive environment" has had a significant impact on the way psychiatric nursing is practiced. Key to nursing care is the therapeutic nurse-client relationship (which can be loosely defined as a genuine desire to help the client coupled with the practice of effective communication techniques and the demonstration of respect for the independence of the client). Communication is much more open and bi-directional now, necessitating a contract between clients and nurses where clients are better informed regarding their conditions and participate more fully in planning their care.

In 1973 the American Nurses Association developed standards of practice (revised in 1982) to provide a framework for psychiatric nursing practice. This evolved in 1994 to the two-part document *"Statement on Psychiatric-Mental Health Clinical Nursing Practice"* and *"Standards of Psychiatric-Mental Health Clinical Practice."* These practice guidelines allow for the standardization of nursing care in all mental health care settings. Since 1988, the American Nurses Credentialing Center has provided nurses with an opportunity to obtain specialty certification as generalists or clinical specialists in psychiatric/mental health nursing through a certification examination (generalist or undergraduate level), or through a combination of clinical supervision, professional recommendations, and an examination (clinical specialist or graduate level). A nurse who practices at the graduate level in the United States may now apply for prescriptive privileges. The breadth and scope of prescribing rules vary depending upon the state in which privileges are granted.

This course will examine broad categories of psychiatric disorders utilizing the guidelines of the *Diagnostic and Statistical Manual of Mental Disorders,* 4th ed., *Text Revision (DSM-IV-TR),* (American Psychiatric Association, 2002). Both adult and child disorders are reviewed, with attention placed on the more commonly encountered diagnoses. Practical applications are emphasized. In most chapters, a case study will be presented and the reader will be provided with a sample nursing care plan, which will include nursing diagnoses, objectives, and interventions. Information on current treatment modalities and medications also will be provided. Chapter objectives and pretest/posttest questions will be used to measure the level of understanding of the reader.

This course is designed for the practicing Registered Nurse (RN) or Licensed Practical/ Vocational Nurse (LPN/LVN). A basic understanding of medical terminology, some abbreviations, and fundamental nursing care is assumed. This course will also be of benefit to the junior or senior nursing student with a particular interest in mental health care. Non-psychiatric nurses who are practicing in an advanced role (e.g., Nurse Practitioners) may find the sections on diagnosing and medication options to be of particular interest.

CHAPTER 1

HISTORY OF MENTAL HEALTH CARE

CHAPTER OBJECTIVE

At the end of this chapter, the reader will be able to discuss the epidemiology and history of mental health care and the diagnosing of psychiatric disorders.

LEARNING OBJECTIVES

At the completion of this chapter, the reader will be able to

1. discuss epidemiological data in prevalence rates of psychiatric disorders, based on information gathered by the National Institute of Mental Health.

2. identify key trends in mental health care over the past century.

3. describe the *DSM-IV-TR* guidelines and how they are utilized in diagnosing psychiatric disorders.

4. define functionality and recognize predictors of a positive outcome in improving functional levels.

EPIDEMIOLOGY

The National Institute of Mental Health (NIMH) estimates that 22.1% of American adults experience a diagnosable psychiatric illness at some point in their life. Nearly 10% of adults develop a depressive disorder with rates two times higher for women than for men. Also twice as high in women are rates for anxiety disorders, which occur in approximately 13.3% of the general population. Bipolar mood disorders affect 2.3 million individuals with women and men equally affected. One out of every 100 persons in the United States suffers from schizophrenia, a chronic and disabling condition, with equal rates for gender. In children and adolescents, approximately 4.1% are diagnosed with attention-deficit/hyperactivity disorder (ADHD). In other words, in a typical American classroom with an average of 25 students, at least one will meet the clinical criteria for ADHD. Cases are 2-3 times higher in boys than in girls. The reverse is true in eating disorders where only 5-15% of clients with an eating disorder are male. The rates of anorexia nervosa in young women are around 3.7%, with 1.1% for bulimia nervosa. The mortality rate among people with anorexia nervosa is approximately 12 times higher than the death rate annually due to all causes in young women. Suicide has been identified as the third leading cause of death in 15- to 24-year-olds (National Institute of Mental Health, 2002).

The last U.S. Census Bureau report dated July 11, 2001, and based on data gathered in 1997, identified approximately 14.3 million Americans on disability for a mental disorder (including dementia) and 3.5 million persons with a learning disability. A disability is defined as difficulty in performing functional tasks or daily living activities. To qualify as a mental disability, the symptoms must seriously interfere with the performance of everyday activities (U.S. Census Bureau, 2001). Data gathered in the 2000 Census Bureau report are scheduled for publication at a later date.

HISTORY OF MENTAL HEALTH CARE

In the late 1700s, the mentally ill were perceived as little better than wild animals. Banishment and confinement were common practices. While families were occasionally provided some assistance by the community, in most cases those with psychiatric disorders were left to wander and fend for themselves. Until 1770, a small fee was charged to visitors of St. Mary of Bethlem Hospital (Bedlam) in England to view the patients. "Treatments" were torturous in nature and included forced feedings, purging, bleeding, and whipping. According to Keltner, et al. (2003), four distinct periods have emerged as benchmarks in the way the mentally ill have been treated since the mid-eighteenth century: moral (or humane) treatment, the age of scientific reason, neurobiological treatment, and deinstitutionalization.

When Philippe Pinel became superintendent of two separate institutions (one for men and one for women) in France in 1793, he noted the deplorable conditions and brutality of the attendants. He unchained clients and brought them out into the sunshine. Simultaneously, William Tuke in England was planning a private facility that would ensure "moral treatment" based on Quaker teachings. He saw his facility as a refuge, a place of asylum or safety. In the United States, Boston schoolteacher Dorothea Dix was instrumental in helping to open 32 state hospitals advocating warmth, food, and protection for residents. A movement toward seeing the mentally ill as human beings with rights to dignity had begun.

The second major shift in the way mental illness was perceived occurred 80 years later during the age of "scientific reason." Sigmund Freud began talking about the influence of early childhood experiences in shaping the psyche. Freud's work stimulated many to follow (Carl Jung, Alfred Adler, and others) providing models of care that are still used today. Emil Kraepelin was the first to describe, classify, and label distinct mental disorders. Other theorists emerged making major contributions in the fields of behaviorism (Watson, Pavlov), somatic treatment (psychosurgery, electroconvulsive therapy, insulin shock), and biology. During this period, individuals with psychiatric disorders could finally receive medical care along with rehabilitative treatment.

In the 1950s, the third benchmark period evolved with the discovery of psychotropic medications. Chlorpromazine (Thorazine®) was the first such agent. Lithium and imipramine (Tofranil®) were identified a few years later. Prior to the discovery and synthesis of chlorpromazine, various concoctions were used to calm clients. These often contained dangerous combinations of alcohol, barbiturates, or opiates. Chlorpromazine was different in that the actual symptoms of the illnesses remitted in many clients. Lithium was accidentally discovered to ameliorate rapid and severe mood swings in clients during the study of its usefulness in epilepsy. It rapidly became a state-of-the-art medication for bipolar illness. Imipramine, a tricyclic antidepressant, was the first medication with treatment efficacy for clinical depression. It has since demonstrated usefulness in the treatment of anxiety and ADHD as well. Monoamine oxidase inhibitors followed tricyclic antidepressants in the treatment of depression. With the availability of effective medications, a gradual shift in perspective among the public occurred. Clients were increasingly perceived as suffering from chemical imbalances or other, as yet unknown, physical defects that hopefully could be corrected through medical treatment.

The Community Mental Health Centers (CMHC) Act of 1963 initiated a trend to remove psychiatric inpatients from hospitals and return them to their home communities. This "deinstitutionalization" benchmark period began when state hospitals had reached their peak census population in 1955. After the CMHC Act, federal legislation provided mentally ill persons with an income by providing definitions for disability and financial aid. This aid is now called Supplemental Security Income (SSI) and Social Security Disability Income (SSDI). Public law discontinued these benefits to individuals suffering exclusively from a drug or alcohol addiction in 1997. Finally, changes in involuntary commitment laws made it more difficult for individuals to be hospitalized unless there were specific criteria met indicating the person was a danger to him or herself, or unable to provide for basic needs of food, shelter, and self-care. These changes were difficult for communities to accept primarily based on fear of the mentally ill, but also on concerns over a potential increase in homelessness and crime. Community-based, regional centers were developed whose primary purpose was to provide care for deinstitutionalized individuals and manage some of these public concerns. Today hundreds of community mental health care centers are located throughout the United States, divided regionally. Each of these centers is charged with the task of assisting adults and children with chronic psychiatric, behavioral, or addictive disorders in maintaining their function within the community in which they reside.

THE DIFFICULTY OF DIAGNOSING AND THE *DSM-IV-TR*

Identifying and diagnosing a psychiatric disorder has always been a difficult task. Unlike most physical health disorders, blood tests cannot reveal a psychiatric illness and are primarily useful in ruling out other diagnoses. X-rays, computerized tomography (CAT) scans, and magnetic resonance imaging (MRI) are only useful in identifying vascular or structural changes in the brain. Recently, positive emission tomography (PET) scans have been studied as a means of identifying some individuals with brain-based disorders. Early research with PET scans looks promising, with changes demonstrated in both the level of brain activity and physical structure in individuals with schizophrenia, but the clinical value of this testing is currently indeterminate. Indirect measures have been practiced for years, notably 24-hour urine collections to evaluate serotonin breakdown in the form of 5HT excretion, and the dexamethasone suppression test to indicate depression syndromes, but these are unreliable and difficult to administer. Additionally, clinicians have varied in their descriptions of psychiatric disorders and there has historically been a lack of common language for the psychiatric care provider.

Kraepelin was one of the first clinicians to develop a set of criteria that could be used in differentiating various symptoms of psychiatric disorders and placing them into some type of categorization. In the United States, the need to collect statistical information resulted in early definitions of mental illnesses. "Idiocy/insanity" was the terminology utilized in the 1840 census. By 1880, seven categories were identified — mania, melancholia, monomania, paresis, dementia, dipsomania, and epilepsy. In 1917, the Committee on Statistics of the American Medico-Psychological Association (later renamed the American Psychiatric Association) developed a plan for the Bureau of Census for gathering uniform statistics by identifying nationally acceptable nomenclature to label mental disorders. Following World War II, the U.S. Army and Veteran's Administration expanded on these diagnostic categories to better incorporate the types of problems experienced by veterans. Around the same time, the World Health Organization (WHO) published the sixth edition of the *International Classification of Diseases* (ICD-6). A variation of the *ICD-6* was published in 1952 by the American Psychiatric Association (APA) and was the first edition of the *Diagnostic and Statistical Manual of Mental Disorders* (DSM-I). Revisions and new additions occurred every 5-10 years to the present date. In 1994, the *DSM-IV* was published as the preeminent classification system for diagnosing and describing psychiatric disorders. More than 1,000 people, in 15 task groups, conducted a 3-stage empirical process that included comprehensive reviews of the published literature, reexamination of existing data sets, and extensive field trials (which collected information on the reliability and characteristics of each criteria set). As the information in the text runs the risk of becoming increasingly outdated with each passing year and each new research study, a text revision was undertaken in 2000. No substantive changes in the criteria sets were done, neither was there any addition of new disorders or subtypes.

Since 2002, the *Diagnostic and Statistical Manual of Mental Disorders,* 4th Edition, *Text Revision* (DSM-IV-TR) has been the primary educational and resource tool for evaluating and categorizing psychiatric disorders. The *ICD-10* was published by the WHO in 1992 (although to date the *ICD-9* is still utilized) and is fully coordinated with the *DSM-IV-TR* in codes and terms used. In the *DSM-IV-TR,* "mental disorders" is defined as a "clinically significant behavioral or psychological syndrome or pattern that occurs in an individual and that is associated with present distress (e.g., a painful symptom) or disability (i.e., impairment in one or more important areas of functioning) or with a significantly increased risk of suffering death, pain, disability, or an important loss of freedom," (*DSM-IV-TR,* 2002). The manual goes on to say "that in order to be identified as a 'mental disorder,'

the syndrome or pattern cannot be an expectable or culturally sanctioned response to an event such as bereavement seen after a death. 'Mental disorders' are psychological/biological and cannot be socially deviant behaviors or conflicts between the individual and society.''

The *DSM-IV-TR* is limited by its use of categorical classifications. Individuals vary in their symptoms and most don't fit neatly into one specific category. The diagnostic criteria provided should be utilized by trained clinicians and serve as a guideline to assist in making sound clinical decisions. Diagnosing does not imply etiology — therefore using the *DSM-IV-TR* to predict dangerousness or future behaviors is inappropriate. The disorders covered in this text will utilize criteria and definitions provided in the *DSM-IV-TR*.

Efforts were made to incorporate cultural awareness into the *DSM-IV-TR* due to the extent of diverse populations seen in today's health care setting. A clinician must have an awareness of culturally appropriate behaviors in order to avoid mislabeling a particular behavior as symptomatic of a mental disorder. The *DSM-IV-TR* contains information to aid mental health care professionals in making culturally sensitive evaluations including: 1) a discussion of cultural variations within clinical presentations; 2) a description of culture-bound syndromes; 3) an outline for cultural formulation to assist the clinician in systematically evaluating the impact of the client's cultural context.

Lastly, the *DSM-IV-TR* is organized in a 5-axis format. Axis I consists of primary psychiatric disorders, which are diagnosed by comparing patient symptoms to a set of standardized criteria. In most cases, the client must meet a minimum number of criteria (e.g., 4 out of 6) in order to receive a specific diagnosis. Axis I may have one or many diagnoses, and they may include other issues important to treatment such as traumatic life events or impaired marital relationships. Axis II is specific to aspects of the client's psyche that impact on the primary psychiatric disorders, specifically personality type disorders or mental retardation. Axis III refers to all medical conditions (which may or may not impact on the psychiatric condition). Axis IV is the clinician's assessment of the type and level of stress clients experience in their social environment, which may worsen or ameliorate the psychiatric disorder(s). Finally, Axis V is a standardized Global Assessment of Functioning (GAF) scale numbering 1-100 that the clinician utilizes to assign a number rating to client on how they react to items noted in Axes I-IV. This number is a useful tool for assessing outcomes as well as evaluating the degree of psychiatric impairment and safety risk.

Example of Diagnosing Utilizing the *DSM-IV-TR* Format:

Adult Client

Axis I:	Schizophrenia, paranoid type, Polysubstance dependence
Axis II:	No diagnosis
Axis III:	Morbid obesity, hypertension, Type II Diabetes mellitus
Axis IV:	Moderate — problems with finances, lack of social support
Axis V:	Current GAF — 48

Child Client

Axis I:	Posttraumatic stress disorder, Reactive attachment disorder, Phonological disorder
Axis II:	Mild mental retardation
Axis III:	Mild intermittent asthma
Axis IV:	Severe — foster home placement (3rd in 2 years), school failure
Axis V:	Current GAF — 55

PREDICTORS OF A POSITIVE OUTCOME

Positive outcomes consist of an increase in the overall functional level of the individual while minimizing detrimental symptoms and excessive resource utilization (cost). Keep in mind that what is perceived as desirable in an adult client, may appear to be different than that of a young child; however, some basic similarities clearly exist. For example, adults are expected to be able to participate in and contribute to society in productive ways such as paid employment, volunteer work, or caring for a family. When an adult experiences a severe and disabling condition, this role performance is threatened. Whereas children only have expectations that they will participate in the learning experience through education, and be a fully involved member of the family and future member of society. Both populations benefit from healthy peer interactions and social relationships at a level considered developmentally appropriate. Clearly, a reduction in physical impairments and risk factors for serious physical and mental illnesses is another standard by which one can measure good health. Chronic mental illness impacts on all aspects of an individual's life. The field of psychiatric medicine is vigorously researching means to alleviate negative symptoms and provide safe and effective medical intervention for individuals. Other mental health care providers are challenged with the task of examining their client's functional levels and problem areas, and working with them to identify interventions that will promote a maximum level of independence, good health, and happiness.

Negative outcomes cost society a great deal — not only in money spent on hospitalization or incarceration, but also in the loss of productive contributions that individuals may be capable of making in their lifetime. Some predictors have been identified that are associated with higher relapse rates, frequent emergency department visits, more frequent and longer inpatient stays, incarceration, violence, or homelessness. A study of 1,456 low-income, adult patients in California (Silver & Holman, 2000), found that the personal experience of a trauma was significantly correlated with higher incidences of psychiatric disturbance. The study defined trauma in four ways: personal violence or witnessing violence outside of the home, including physical or sexual assault; domestic violence; witnessing death; and acute loss or accident. The Treatment Advocacy Center of Arlington, VA, reported in their 2002 Fact Sheet that primary predictors of violence included a history of past violence, the presence of drug or alcohol abuse, and medication noncompliance in a person with a serious brain disorder. They also identified potential violence predictors as the presence of command hallucinations, paranoid delusions, and significant neurological impairments.

Treatment providers can intervene in a number of ways to reduce the risk of relapse. Encouraging clients to participate in self-help groups, especially when drugs or alcohol are involved, has been consistently shown to positively impact on psychiatric stability. Advocacy and support through organizations such as the National Alliance for the Mentally Ill (NAMI) or Children and Adults with Attention Deficit Disorder (CHADD) is recommended for family members and clients alike. In a 2000 study of inmates in Florida, researchers found that active case management reduced the length of stay in an acute psychiatric care facility by as much as 27% (Bedard & DeVolentine, 2000).

A number of reports compiled by Gabbard & Lazar for the American Psychiatric Association Commission on Psychotherapy by Psychiatrists (2002) found that psychotherapy sessions reduced hospitalizations, medical expenses, and overall work disability.

Psychiatric nurses can have a significant impact in mental health care promotion and disease prevention through educating clients and their families, encouraging self-help and advocacy programs, providing case management, monitoring medication administration and efficacy, and providing direct care. Psychiatric nurses are in a unique position in the multidisciplinary health care team of viewing "whole" clients and their support systems, and being able to facilitate care planning in a manner designed to restore clients to an optimal level of functioning, both for their own well being and to the benefit of society in general.

EXAM QUESTIONS

CHAPTER 1
Questions 1-8

1. The percentage of adults who will meet the clinical criteria for depression at some point in their lives is
   a. 10%.
   b. 20%.
   c. 30%.
   d. 40%.

2. The major shift in the perception of mental illness as a medical disorder is known as the age of
   a. religious exorcisms.
   b. shunning.
   c. home-based care.
   d. scientific reason.

3. The government action that initiated deinstitutionalization was the
   a. Supplemental Security Income & Social Security Disability Income Legislation.
   b. Community Mental Health Centers Act.
   c. Statement on Psychiatric-Mental Health Clinical Nursing Practice Standard.
   d. Certification of Generalist and Specialist Psychiatric Nurses.

4. The benchmark period associated with bringing patients out of hospitals and into the fresh air and sunshine was
   a. moral treatment.
   b. scientific reason.
   c. deinstitutionalization.
   d. neurobiological treatment.

5. The *DSM-IV-TR*
   a. does not address cultural variations.
   b. contains information to aid in making culturally sensitive evaluations.
   c. is only relevant to diagnosing U.S. citizens.
   d. is a culturally-biased tool.

6. The *DSM-IV-TR* utilizes a 5-Axis format. Axis-IV represents
   a. the degree of social stress experienced by the client.
   b. the primary psychiatric diagnosis.
   c. the client's medical diagnosis.
   d. personality and basic character traits.

7. Role performance expectations that are important in childhood include
   a. maintaining a household and caring for siblings.
   b. volunteering for community organizations.
   c. participating in the national economy through paid employment.
   d. participating in the learning experience through education.

8. One predictor of higher psychiatric illness relapse rates is
   a. frequent emergency department visits.
   b. a lack of health care insurance.
   c. frequent medication adjustments.
   d. poor physical health.

CHAPTER 2

ETHICS, LAW, AND CULTURAL VARIATIONS

CHAPTER OBJECTIVE

At the end of this chapter the reader will be able to discuss some of the ethical, legal, and cultural issues associated with mental health care and treatment.

LEARNING OBJECTIVES

At the completion of this chapter, the reader will be able to

1. discuss the role of ethics in mental health care.

2. differentiate between voluntary and involuntary clients.

3. verbalize the importance of maintaining confidentiality and when it may be necessary to break confidentiality.

4. examine cultural differences as related to mental health care in minority populations in the United States.

ETHICAL PRINCIPLES AND BEHAVIORS

Ethics refers to the beliefs about right and wrong in a person, and the standards of right or wrong in a society. Ethical standards may or may not be consistent with societal norms or laws. Nurses need to have a thorough understanding of general ethical principles in order to make reason-

able, fair, and sound judgments in providing care. Ethical principles cause us to look at how we act in relationships, and how we live with one another. Nurses who choose to work in the field of mental health care will encounter ethical questions on nearly a daily basis. Issues such as confidentiality, patient protection, therapeutic relationships, clinical competency, and mental health research are particularly complicated. To better guide the nurse in making ethical choices, an understanding of general principles will be useful.

General ethical principles fall into five broad categories. The American Psychological Association's Ethics Office discusses these at length on their Web site, www.apa.org/ethics (APAOnline: Ethics Information, 2003). Principles are meant to be guidelines to help the health care provider in decision-making.

1. Beneficence and Nonmaleficence — Health care providers must have the desire to be professional and help the client, and in doing so to "do no harm." The nurse should guard against using undue influence to pressure the client into desired actions. Medication compliance is a good example of where decisions are frequently made that present ethical dilemmas. The health care provider must weigh the pros and cons of administering antipsychotic medications against a client's will in order to address the greater good of ameliorating the psychotic condition or protecting society.

Involuntary treatment may be necessary to both benefit the client, and to prevent future harm.

2. Fidelity and Responsibility — Health care providers have a duty to be honest and trustworthy with their clients. The inherent power in the relationship lies with the caregiver. Clients are asked to be trusting and to believe that others have their best interest in mind. This ascribes a high degree of responsibility on the health care provider to tell the truth and to be accountable for professional behaviors. Ethical issues often arise regarding clinical research and informed consent.

3. Integrity — Health care providers must be professional and maintain a high level of clinical expertise. Nurses practicing in psychiatric settings should obtain continuing education in the mental health field and maintain a certain level of competency. Health care providers must also guard against establishing personal or sexual relationships with clients. In most settings, psychiatric staff members are not permitted to engage in any commerce (buying or selling) with clients for an extended period of time to avoid the appearance of impropriety, or accusations that the staff member is "taking advantage" of the dependent nature of the staff-client relationship.

4. Justice — Health care providers must recognize that all persons are entitled to equal treatment and quality of care, even in the mental health realm. It can be particularly difficult to provide emotional support and counseling equally to both the family harmed by an intoxicated driver, and to the driver himself. Health care providers should strive to be nonjudgmental and fair to all clients regardless of age, gender, race, sexual orientation, diagnosis, or any other differentiating characteristic.

5. Respect — Health care providers need to respect the dignity and worth of all people, and

the rights of individuals to confidentiality, privacy, and freedom of choice. The psychiatric nurse should also respect religious and cultural differences and strive to avoid ethnocentrism. Clients experiencing an acute exacerbation of a psychiatric disorder may behave oddly or inappropriately at times. The nurse needs to refrain from laughing or otherwise demeaning the client, and protect the client as much as possible from a loss of dignity.

When faced with a difficult decision, it is useful to have a framework for decision-making to guide the health care provider. First, it is important to gather all of the facts of a situation: What is the dilemma? Who will be affected? What are possible outcomes? For each course of action, what may be the result? Are there legal issues at stake? After making a thorough examination of the relevant information, one can next consider alternative actions from various moral perspectives:

The Virtue Perspective

- Identifies moral values as what are inherently positive character traits.

- Includes honesty, faithfulness, integrity, compassion, truthfulness, and courage.

- Decisions are based on what is *the right thing to do.*

The Utilitarian Perspective

- Weighs the effects of actions against the consequence there will be to society. May sacrifice rights of the individual for the greater good.

- Decisions are based on what is *best for the majority.*

The Rights Perspective

- Focuses on the rights of the individual (civil, political) and respects the dignity of the person.

- Includes issues of "right to free speech," "right to liberty," "right to privacy."

- Decisions are based on what *protects basic rights.*

The Fairness (or Justice) Perspective

- States that all must be treated equally and consistently unless there is moral justification for treating some differently (some "deserve" it more).

- Involves moral justification may be based on needs, merit, or faults.

- Decisions are based on *treating based on moral justifications.*

The Common Good Perspective

- Describes that the good of the individual is bound to the common good of the community. The community has shared values and goals.

- Decisions are based on *the advancement of the community.*

The nurse is then faced with making a decision. Decisions do not have to be made alone — in fact, involving the multidisciplinary mental health care team (usually comprised of nursing, medicine, social work, rehabilitation, and psychology) can provide a safety net for the nurse and ensure that personal biases are eliminated.

As a final step, those involved need to reflect on the decision made, actions, and subsequent results. What, if anything, should have been done differently? Were the basic principles of beneficence, fidelity, integrity, justice, and respect maintained? Were goals accomplished? How will these actions influence the client's future care?

Additionally, one should consider the issue of ethical relativism. Ethical relativism deals with the differences in ethical beliefs relative to one's societal norms. An action deemed appropriate or "right" in one culture, may be very unacceptable in another. Some ethicists claim that there is no universal moral standard — all ethics are culture bound and moral standards can only be determined within a specific society — while others believe that fundamental principles exist in all cultures and are inherent in all human beings. Consider the act of infanticide. American culture treats the killing of infants equal to the killing of any person while other cultures have practiced infanticide when obvious birth defects are present, or starvation of other children is at risk. Relativism is also evident on a historical basis. Hundreds of years ago, intermarriage with first cousins and even siblings (royalty) was encouraged to maintain the family bloodlines. Today it is unacceptable in most parts of the world.

LEGAL CONSIDERATIONS: VOLUNTARY VERSUS INVOLUNTARY CLIENTS

In Section 1 of the 14th Amendment of the U.S. Constitution it states that, "All persons born or naturalized in the United States, and subject to the jurisdiction thereof, are citizens of the United States and of the state wherein they reside. No state shall…deprive any person of life, liberty, or property, without due process of law; nor deny to any person within its jurisdiction the equal protection of the laws."

The issue of liberty has been tested repeatedly in settings where U.S. citizens have been held against their will, including psychiatric institutions.

Keltner, Schwecke, & Bostrom (2003) do an excellent job of providing an overview of landmark legal decisions related to individuals with a psychiatric disorder. They identify 10 rulings that have historically made a marked impact on the legal right of both the identified clients, and on affected other parties. A summary of these legal decisions follows:

1. 1843 — The *M'Naghten rule* first identified a legal defense of "not guilty by reason of insanity" by stating that persons who do not understand the nature of their actions cannot be held legally responsible for those actions.

2. 1965 — In *Griswold v. Connecticut* the U.S. Supreme Court first recognized that an individual has a "right of personal privacy" under the Constitution of the United States.

3. 1966 — *Rouse v. Cameron* was a case where the courts found that a person committed to an institution must be actively receiving treatment and not merely warehoused.

4. 1968 — *Whitree v. State of New York* was a case where a client who had been institutionalized for 14 years successfully sued the state of New York claiming that if he had received adequate treatment he could have been discharged after only 2 years.

5. 1968 — In *Meier v. Ross General Hospital*, a physician was found liable for the death of his hospitalized client who committed suicide while under his care. The client had a previous suicide attempt prior to the hospital stay. The physician was liable for failing in his "duty to warn" of the threat of suicide in this client.

6. 1972 — In *Wyatt v. Stickney*, the entire mental health care system of Alabama was sued for an inadequate treatment program. The court ruled that each institution within the mental health care system must: a) stop using clients for hospital labor needs, b) ensure a humane environment, c) maintain minimum staffing levels, d) establish human rights committees, and e) provide the least restrictive environment possible for the client.

7. 1976 — In the well-known case of *Tarakoff v. The Regents of the University of California*, the parents of Tatiana Tarakoff sued the university following the 1969 death of their daughter at the hands of Prosenjit Poddar. Poddar had told his therapist that he planned to kill Tarakoff when she returned from summer break. Although the therapist had contacted the police, they released Poddar because he appeared rational. The court found that the therapist had a "duty to warn of threats of harm to others" and was negligent in not notifying Tarakoff of the threats that had been made against her.

8. 1979 — Clients at Boston State Hospital sought the "right to refuse treatment" in *Rogers v. Okin*. Based on the 1965 decision regarding the "right of personal privacy," the court found that the hospital could not force nonviolent clients to take medication against their will. This ruling also included the directive that clients or their guardians must give informed consent before medications could be given.

9. 1983 — In *Rennie v. Klein*, a client claimed his rights were violated by the hospital when he was forced to take psychotropic medications. The ruling again addressed the "right to refuse treatment" and the "right to privacy," and furthered the necessity of obtaining informed consent.

10. 1972 — *Jackson v. Indiana*, and 1992 — *Foucha v. Louisiana*, both demonstrated that the nature of a (ongoing) psychiatric commitment must "bear some reasonable relation to the purpose for which the individual is committed" (Justice White of the Supreme Court). When Jackson and Foucha were first hospitalized, they were deemed to be mentally ill and dangerous. The ruling recognized that individuals who are no longer mentally ill do not require hospitalization, and that individuals are not required to prove themselves to be no longer dangerous.

THE BAKER ACT

In 1971, the legislature of Florida adopted the Florida Mental Health Act (The Baker Act), thus dramatically revising and updating almost 100 years of mental health involuntary commitment practice. The Baker Act was named after Maxine Baker, former state representative from Miami who sponsored the act after serving as chairperson of the House Committee on Mental Health. The overall purpose of the Baker Act was to systematically address the limitations on liberty placed upon an individual with a psychiatric disorder. The Baker

Act has since been revised with its most recent reform occurring in 1996 to further reinforce, among other things, protection for voluntarily admitted clients, clients being released from state treatment facilities, informed consent and guardian advocacy, and expanded notice requirements (McGaha & Stiles, 2001).

The Baker Act is broad in its coverage. It ensures that individuals be treated humanely and fairly and includes the rights to send and receive mail and telephone calls, to keep one's own possessions and clothing, and the right to register and vote in public elections. It guarantees clients the right to have visitors when requested and covers the right to receive appropriate treatment, or to refuse treatment. Use of restraints, seclusion, isolation, and other management techniques are closely monitored and complaint resolution is required. The Baker Act ensures that clients have the right to ask the court to review the cause and legality of any detention of unjust denial of a right or privilege or authorized procedure. Additionally, the client has the right to participate in treatment and discharge planning, seeking out the practitioner of choice. In any instance where these rights are denied, the health care providers must be able to thoroughly document the rationale for the denial and notify the client, preferably in writing. The health care provider may never restrict telephone calls to the client's attorney.

An admission to a psychiatric facility differs from a medical facility in that there must be a clear (not implied) legal status of the client. Preferentially, all hospitalized clients are admitted voluntarily and have agreed, in writing, to receiving inpatient care. The client must be informed of the reason for admission, and purpose of the proposed treatment, as well as the approximate length of care and side effects that may be incurred as a result of treatment prior to being admitted. Adults must be deemed mentally competent to give their consent. A minor child may only be admitted to a

psychiatric facility upon the application and signature of a legal guardian. Occasionally, a voluntarily admitted client will decide to leave the hospital against medical or clinical advice. The attending physician must determine whether the client's thoughts or behaviors will constitute a danger to himself, or a danger to others, or whether the client is so gravely ill that he will be unable to provide for basic needs of food, shelter, clothing, and protection from the elements. If the determination is made that the client is not safe to leave the facility, then involuntary commitment proceedings are initiated. This decision must be made within 24 hours of the client's request to be discharged.

Particular care must be taken when hospitalizing an adult client with a dementia disorder, or who has a health care surrogate or proxy, to a psychiatric facility. Prior to the admission, these clients must be assessed as to their ability to provide informed consent for the admission. If there is a question as to the competency of the client, it may be preferable to refuse a voluntary admission and obtain a court order for an involuntary examination. A competency hearing may also be necessary.

Clients may be evaluated on an involuntary basis when they refuse voluntary treatment (or if they are not competent to consent to voluntary treatment). Without care or treatment, clients are likely to suffer from neglect. This can result in a real and present threat to the self, with a substantial likelihood that serious bodily harm may be caused to the self or others in the near future. An involuntary examination may be requested, or petitioned, by any concerned party (usually a family member), and must be initiated by one of the following: a court may enter an ex parte order based upon sworn testimony; a law enforcement officer may take the client into custody and deliver him to a treatment facility; or a physician, clinical psychologist, psychiatric nurse, or clinical social worker may execute a certificate stating that the client has been examined within the past 48 hours and found to meet the criteria for involuntary examination, after which a court will issue an order to admit the client involuntarily to the nearest accepting treatment facility. Once an involuntary examination has been initiated, the receiving facility has 72 working hours (does not include weekends or legal holidays) to examine the client and determine whether psychiatric treatment is required. At the end of the 72 hours, the client must be released (to outpatient care, unless charged with a crime, then to the appropriate police department) or sign a voluntary admission application, or the attending physician must petition the court for involuntary placement.

An involuntary placement may be ordered by the court when there is clear and convincing evidence that the client suffers from a mental illness, *and* has refused voluntary treatment (or is unable to decide), *and* without the placement a real and present threat of substantial harm to the clients' well-being exists; *or* without the placement there is a substantial likelihood that the client will inflict self-harm, or harm others, *and* all available less-restrictive treatment alternatives have been deemed inappropriate. The court then states the length of time that the client will be under an involuntary placement order. At the end of this time, the health care team must decide whether to pursue continued involuntary placement.

Psychiatric nurses should become familiar with their individual state laws that govern the specifics of voluntary and involuntary psychiatric admissions, as well as the procedures followed by specific health care facilities. It is not unusual to find variations on the interpretation of the Baker Act from state to state or in different regions of the country.

CONFIDENTIALITY AND THE BILL OF RIGHTS

In 1998, President Clinton appointed the Advisory Commission on Consumer Protection and Quality in the Health Care Industry. The Commission, co-chaired by Donna Shalala, secretary of the Department of Health and Human Services, issued its final report that included a Consumer Bill of Rights and Responsibilities (see Table 2-1). Of particular interest to psychiatric nurses is the section on confidentiality of health information. Psychiatric clients are expressly protected in the confidentiality of their records; information may not be shared with any third-party without the express written consent of the client or his legal guardian. Consent to release information may be withdrawn at any time by the client. Few exceptions to this exist. Confidentiality may be violated only in these situations

1. The client has made a direct threat against another person, and the health care provider has a clear "duty to warn" the endangered individual.

2. The client has reported actual or suspected abuse (including molestation) or neglect of a minor child. The health care provider has an obligation to report this to the appropriate Child Protective Services division of the state Office of Family and Children.

3. The health care provider may discuss the information provided in a commitment document with the relevant physician, officer of the court, and petitioner(s) of the commitment.

4. When an insanity defense is utilized to defend against a criminal charge, the entire clinical record becomes public.

5. A judge may order documents (clinical records) to be turned over to the court for examination. A subpoena to appear in court does not constitute a judge's order to release information, merely it mandates the appearance of the subpoenaed individual.

Violation of the confidentiality of a psychiatric client in situations other than those outlined herein may subject the nurse to legal action as well as licensure

TABLE 2-1: CONSUMER BILL OF RIGHTS AND RESPONSIBILITIES

I. *Information Disclosure* — You have the right to receive accurate and easily understood information about your health plan, health care professionals, and health care facilities. If you speak another language, have a physical or mental disability, or just don't understand something, assistance will be provided so you can make informed health care decisions.

II. *Choice of Providers and Plans* — You have the right to a choice of health care providers that is sufficient to provide you with access to appropriate high-quality health care.

III. *Access to Emergency Services* — If you have severe pain, an injury, or sudden illness that convinces you that your health is in serious jeopardy, you have the right to receive screening and stabilization emergency services whenever and wherever needed, without prior authorization or financial penalty.

IV. *Participation in Treatment Decisions* — You have the right to know all your treatment options and to participate in decisions about your care. Parents, guardians, members, or other individuals that you designate can represent you if you cannot make your own decisions.

V. *Respect and Nondiscrimination* — You have the right to considerate, respectful and nondiscriminatory care from your doctors, health plan representatives, and other health care providers.

VI. *Confidentiality of Health Information* — You have the right to talk in confidence with health care providers and to have your health care information protected. You also have the right to review and copy your own medical record and request that your physician amend your record if it is not accurate, relevant, or complete.

VII. *Complaints and Appeals* — You have the right to a fair, fast and objective review of any complaint you have against your health plan, doctors, hospitals or other health care personnel. This includes complaints about waiting times, operating hours, the conduct of health care personnel, and the adequacy of health care facilities.

Note. From MEDLINEplus Medical Encyclopedia: Consumer rights and responsibilities. (November 23, 2002). Available at: www.nlm.nih.gov/medlineplus/ency/article/001947.htm, a service of the U.S. National Library of Medicine and the National Institutes of Health.

censure. Most agencies have an acceptable form that identifies to whom information may be released, date that the release is valid, and particular types of information that can be shared. In 2003, the Health Insurance Protection and Portability Act (HIPPA) went into effect. This act is designed to protect client information more securely with the advent of various forms of electronic data submission and documentation.

CULTURAL DIVERSITY ISSUES

Culture influences various aspects of mental health including the recognition and expression of psychiatric symptoms, coping styles, community supports, and the willingness to seek treatment. Culture-bound syndromes are recurrent, locality-specific patterns of aberrant behavior that are not linked to a specific *DSM-IV-TR* diagnostic category. Most of these are limited to specific ethnic populations and are, in essence, diagnostic categories used to identify, discuss, and treat specific problem behaviors or symptoms within that culture. Appendix A examines some culture-bound syndromes identified in the *DSM-IV-TR* along with characteristic traits of each syndrome.

In 1999, the U.S. Department of Health and Human Services, Office of the Surgeon General, collected data on the mental health of various cultures and ethnic populations in the United States.

Four primary ethnicities were studied: African Americans, Asian American/Pacific Islanders, Latinos/Hispanic Americans, and Native American Indians/Alaska Natives. Table 2-2 presents a summary of demographic differences identified in these populations as compared to the general population of all U.S. citizens. Mental health problems including depression, posttraumatic stress disorder and alcoholism have long been associated with social problem of poverty, homelessness, poor education, and incarceration.

African Americans constitute approximately 12% of the U.S. population. In 1999, 22% lived below poverty guidelines. Mental health providers are predominately not African American, with only about 2% of psychiatrists and psychologists, and

4% of social workers represented. Few clinical trials have focused primarily on the African American population. Limited data suggests that mental health rates are the same for all ethnic groups, but there is alarming cause for concerns in diagnostic accuracy. African Americans are more likely than Whites to be diagnosed with schizophrenia, and less likely than whites to be diagnosed or treated for depression. Additionally, African Americans are more likely to be treated in hospital settings, and less likely to receive outpatient services. Older African Americans (especially women) were found to enter post-hospital home care with higher levels of physical and cognitive impairments, and to have caregivers with more limitations than did older Whites. Older African American adults may also be reluctant to share

TABLE 2-2: SOCIAL DEMOGRAPHICS OF CULTURAL MINORITIES IN THE UNITED STATES

Population	% of all U.S. Citizens	% with High School Education - Compared to Total U.S. Populations	% Living at or Below Poverty - Compared to Total U.S. Population	% Incarcerated - Compared to Total U.S. Incarcerated Population	% Children in the Welfare System - Compared to Total U.S. Children in Welfare System	% Homeless - Compared to Total U.S. Homeless Population
African Americans	12%	*	22%	40-50%	45%	40%
Latino/ Hispanic Americans	12-15%	56%	14-30%	9%	*	*
Asian American/ Pacific Islanders	4%	Variable	14%	*	*	Significantly high in Refugee status
American Indian Native/Alaska Native	1.5%	56%	26%	1 out of every 25 AI/AN adults	1%	8%
Total U.S. Population	100%	83%	13.5%	N/A	100%	100%

Note. From U.S. Department of Health and Human Services, Office of the Surgeon General, SAMHSA. (1999).
* Data not provided in Surgeon General's report.

information with non-African American health care providers due to historical experiences with racism and the belief that they will not be listened to or shown respect.

The Latino/Hispanic American population is rapidly growing. If trends continue, Latinos/ Hispanics will comprise 25% of Americans by the year 2050. Mexican Americans constitute nearly two-thirds of the Hispanic population. Rates of mental health disorders are similar to non-Hispanic Whites with some exceptions: adult immigrants have lower rates of mental disorders than American-born Mexican Americans or Puerto Ricans; Latino youths experience more anxiety and delinquency problems, depression, and drug use than do non-Hispanic White youths; depression in older adults is closely correlated with physical illness; and suicide rates in 1997 were about 50% that of non-Hispanic Whites (although suicide ideation and unsuccessful attempts were higher). There is a higher incidence of posttraumatic stress disorder (PTSD) in Hispanic men — associated with refugees exposed to civil wars in their home countries, and to Vietnam veterans. Substance abuse rates are slightly lower in Hispanic women, and slightly higher in Hispanic men. Hispanics are approximately twice as likely as Whites to die from liver cirrhosis — possibly related to a higher incidence of hepatitis C. There are few Hispanic children in the child welfare system, but Latino men are four times more likely than Whites to be incarcerated at some point in their lifetime. The lack of Spanish-speaking mental health care providers has been a problem, causing fewer than one in 11 individuals with a psychiatric disorder to seek treatment. Misdiagnosing is common related to language barriers. Hispanic Americans are more likely to utilize folk remedies solely, or as a complement to traditional care, and some may consult folk healers for more traditional care. The ill and older people are more likely to be cared for within the home community, partly due to the strength of family values.

Asian Americans/Pacific Islanders (AA/PI) comprise approximately 4% of the U.S. population. There are more than 43 different ethnic subgroups included in the AA/PI category, with over 100 languages and dialects. About 35% live in households where there is limited English proficiency. Mental health care needs have not been well studied in this group. Prevalence rates for depression are around 3-7% using traditional scales. Asian Americans tend to exhibit somatic (physical) complaints of depression more frequently. Culture-bound syndromes may include neurasthenia characterized by fatigue, weakness, poor concentration, memory loss, irritability, aches and pains, sleep disturbances, and Hwa-byung (Appendix A). The focus on physical symptoms can serve as a barrier to seeking mental health care. Older Asian Americans may not understand questions or the intent of a medical interview, and may answer "yes" to avoid confrontation. Suicide rates tend to be lower overall with the exceptions being Native Hawaiian adolescents, and older Asian American women (over age 65). Social isolation may be a factor in higher suicide rates of older adults. Many AA/PI's are heavily represented among refugee populations and, as such, are at higher risk for PTSD — in some studies as high as 70% for Southeast Asian refugees. Nearly 50% of this population will have difficulty in accessing mental health care services because of language barriers. Utilization of mental health care services is extremely low. Shame and stigma are believed to figure prominently in these low utilization rates. The use of complementary therapies (such as herbal) is higher than in the general population. Alcoholism tends to be lower. Many Asian Americans have a decreased activity of the enzyme aldehyde dehydrogenase-2, a necessary component for the metabolism of alcohol. As a result, alcohol tolerance is very low.

In the general population, 1.5% of the population is identified as being of American Indian or

Alaska Native (AI/AN) heritage. There are at least 561 different AI/AN tribes and over 200 indigenous languages. There are no large-scale epidemiological studies examining mental health prevalence or differences to date; however the Great Smoky Mountain Study found that American Indian children were the same as White children in rates of psychiatric disorders with lower rates of tics but higher rates of substance abuse (among 13-year-old children). Suicide rates for AI/ANs are 1.5 times the national average. Alcohol/drug problems are higher than in other populations (up to 70% in Northern Plains Indians). Deaths from chronic liver disease and cirrhosis are about 4 times more prevalent among AI/ANs than in the general U.S. population. Violence exposure and trauma is more than twice the national average with a lifetime prevalence of PTSD in Vietnam veterans as high as 57%. The Indian Health Service (IHS) is the federal agency responsible for providing health care to native populations. Only about 20% of Native American Indians report access to IHS clinics, which are located on reservations. Mental health treatment rates appear to be the same or similar to those of non-American Indian/Alaska Native Whites — about 32% of those with an identified disorder seek treatment. Among Cherokee children, only one in 7 received professional treatment and were more likely than White children to be seen in the juvenile justice system. There is a limited availability of skilled and intermediate long-term care facilities on reservations. In 1999, there were only 15 such facilities among the nearly 300 AI/AN reservations. Health care is more likely to be provided within the home community. AI/AN culture tends to view illness as a natural part of the aging process; thus health care may not be readily sought and there is a greater reliance on native remedies.

Psychiatric disorders are prevalent across all populations regardless of ethnicity; however, there has been little research into specific ethnic groups.

Social and economic factors impact greatly on the mental health of a population. Living in poverty has the most significant negative impact, followed by a lack of education and income. Discrimination and racism adversely affect both health status and the willingness to seek treatment. Stigmas against mental disorders and their treatments are as great or even greater in minority populations as in the general U.S. population, and mistrust of mental health care services has been a major deterrent to treatment.

CHAPTER 2

Questions 9-15

9. Ethical decisions ideally should be made by the

    a. physician.

    b. nurse.

    c. family.

    d. multidisciplinary team.

10. One criterion for an involuntary hospital admission is

    a. refusal to take medications.

    b. illegal acts such as burglary.

    c. alcohol intoxication.

    d. a suicide attempt or threat.

11. An involuntary hospital admission is most likely to be necessary with a

    a. person who is hallucinating but is not making any threats to harm himself or others.

    b. person who is confused and talking about alien invasions, is sleeping on the streets, and is dehydrated and malnourished.

    c. person who is intoxicated and angry with the staff of the emergency department of a hospital.

    d. teenager who is writes a letter to his girlfriend telling her he can't live without her.

12. The Baker Act of 1971 guarantees the right to

    a. smoke in designated hospital rooms.

    b. send and receive mail.

    c. take weekend long passes.

    d. commit suicide if terminally ill.

13. Confidentiality of an individual receiving psychiatric treatment can only be violated without the client's consent when the

    a. police have a warrant to arrest the individual.

    b. client reports physical or sexual abuse of a child.

    c. client's wife is calling for information.

    d. client's employer needs to know how long he will be in treatment.

14. The ethnic group studied in the 1999 Surgeon General's report that is expected to reach 25% of the U.S. population by the year 2050 is

    a. African American.

    b. Latino/Hispanic American.

    c. Asian American/Pacific Islander.

    d. American Indian/Alaska Native.

15. A significant factor that prevents minority populations in the United States from seeking mental health treatment is a

    a. lack of money and transportation to get services.

    b. predominance of highly educated individuals.

    c. lower incidence of psychiatric disorders.

    d. mistrust of non-ethnic mental health care providers and fear of discrimination.

CHAPTER 3

NURSING ASSESSMENTS AND PLANNING CARE

CHAPTER OBJECTIVE

At the end of this chapter, the reader will be able to obtain a nursing history of a psychiatric client and write an effective nursing care plan.

LEARNING OBJECTIVES

At the end of this chapter, the reader will be able to

1. identify key elements of information that need to be obtained in a nursing history.

2. perform a mental status examination.

3. write a nursing care plan with appropriate nursing diagnoses, long-term treatment goals, short-term objectives, and interventions.

THE NURSING PROCESS

The nursing process is a systematic way of approaching the nursing care of an individual experiencing a disruption in health status — whether physical or psychiatric. The nursing process consists of assessment and diagnosis, care planning, carrying out selected interventions, and evaluating the outcome or effectiveness of those interventions. The first crucial step is obtaining a thorough history of the client incorporating elements of the client's current and past health problems, social issues impacting health, and cultural or spiritual beliefs that may support or interfere with prescribed health care treatments.

A nursing history should be obtained in an environment conducive to effective communication between the nurse and the client. Family members and/or significant others may or may not be present, or they may be present for a portion of the time, then be asked to step out to maintain the client's sense of confidentiality. Interviews should be done in a private conference room or client's room (if inpatient or residential) rather than in a public area where others may overhear. If personal safety is a concern, the nurse may request another staff member to be present. Distracting elements such as television or radio should be removed. If the nurse determines that the client is too ill to be able to provide accurate information, or that the interview process itself will be detrimental to the client's health, then information should be obtained from other reliable sources such as family members, social workers, therapists, primary physicians, and so forth. Documentation of the source of information is important, particularly when the client is unable to provide an accurate history.

Most health care facilities will have an existing form to guide the nurse in the collection of data. Appendix B provides an example of a form that incorporates key elements of the nursing history. Whatever format is utilized, the information obtained should readily lead to the development of a problem list. The problem list may be fairly extensive. At this point, the nurse needs to utilize the skill of prioritizing to determine which problems can realistically be addressed given the time and resources available.

Once essential problems have been identified (usually not more than four to six problems depending on the severity of the disorder), the nurse should be prepared to write nursing diagnoses to address the problem(s). Nursing diagnoses are important in structuring the care provided for the client in the most efficient and appropriate manner possible. They also serve as a "common language" between health care providers to better facilitate communication. The North American Nursing Diagnosis Association (NANDA) is an organization that has developed a list of commonly used nursing diagnoses. By utilizing NANDA diagnoses, the nurse can better identify existing or potential problems, contributing factors, and the behavioral expression or symptoms of the disorder (Ackley & Ladwig, 2002). Identifying contributing factors and behavioral symptoms can directly lead to the development of both short-and long-term goals to measure the success of treatment.

Long-term goals are useful in helping the client to determine what the overall desired outcome of care will be. Long-term goals are generally expressed in broad or general terms, and can represent months or even years of treatment. For example, in a depressed client, a long-term goal may be *"The client will have complete symptom remission for a period of one year."* It may be helpful to discuss some of the contributing factors identified in the nursing diagnosis with the client, in order to better understand what elements may interfere with the success of a long-term goal. In the example given, contributing factors could include a lack of prescription medication or health care insurance, which prevents the client from receiving therapy or regular medication treatment. Both long-term and short-term goals are expressed in terms of what the client will be able to achieve.

Short-term goals, often called objectives, are outcome measures that can realistically be achieved during the current course of treatment. These can usually be met within hours, days, or a few weeks. Objectives need to be behavioral in nature. They should be written in such a way that they can be easily measured by the nurse. Verbs such as, "demonstrates," "verbalizes," and "lists," are more appropriate than "knows," "has," or "is" in writing objectives. It is important that the objectives be developed in collaboration with the client so that there is an understanding of what the nurse and other health care providers identify as primary needs. In this way, the client becomes an active part of the health care team. Each nursing diagnosis will lead to at least one objective; more commonly two to four goals or objectives are identified for each diagnosis. Each objective should lead logically to several nursing interventions that are specifically designed to address that objective.

Nursing interventions should be expressed in terms of what the nurse, or other health care providers, will do in order to help the client meet the objectives, and ultimately the long-term goal(s). A statement such as, *"The client will go to A.A. meetings every day,"* is inappropriate, as it is not focused on the health care provider. An appropriate intervention would read, *"Staff will provide transportation to A.A. meetings on a daily basis."* Another common error in writing nursing interventions is that they are often too generalized and vague. Saying a nurse will *"Reorient the client to reality"* doesn't specify how the client will be reoriented, what techniques or tools are needed, or what role each specific health care provider will carry out in the reorientation process. It is more useful for the nurse to select out a smaller number of very specific objectives and nursing interventions that can be understood and attained, than to write a "laundry list" of objectives and interventions that will not realistically be utilized by the health care staff.

The final phase of the nursing process consists of reflecting on the goals and objectives written, and determining whether or not the interventions were effective. This evaluation of care should be systematic and address each of the objectives identified. When objectives are written in very specific, behavioral measures, then it is a simple matter to assess goal attainment. If an objective is, *"The client will demonstrate how to measure and self-administer his insulin accurately every time,"* then the nurse can easily determine if this objective is met at 100%, 50%, or not at all. The final task is to determine what prevented the client from meeting the objectives. Perhaps they were not developed in collaboration with the client. In this case, there were likely unidentified barriers that prevented the objectives from being met. It may be that the objectives set were too vague or could not be met in the time available. Interventions may not have been clear, carried out, or associated with the goals of care. The initial problem identification, prioritization, and nursing diagnosis may not have accurately reflected which problems were primary. A thorough examination of goal attainment will lead the nurse to revise the care plan to more effectively target the problems identified.

MENTAL STATUS EXAMS

Mental Status Exams, or assessments, are a structured means of examining the mental and emotional state of a psychiatric client to better lead to an appropriate diagnosis. They can also point the clinician toward significant problem areas to be targeted in a care plan. Mental status exams are an essential tool for evaluating safety for both the client and the caregivers. Exams may follow many different formats, and most health care facilities will have a form already in place. All exams will include the same basic elements: an examination of the client's behaviors, thoughts, and moods.

Appearance

Overall appearance is the first element assessed in a mental status exam. How is the client groomed? Is their any obvious soiling of the person or clothing? Is there an odor present? Is the client wearing clothing that is appropriate to the weather and environment? It is important to take housing and financial means into consideration, as a client who is homeless or indigent may have less access to stylish clothing or hygiene items than one who lives in a middle-class, suburban setting.

Behavior

The client's behavior during the interview should be noted. Is the client cooperative and maintaining good eye contact? Or, does the client present as evasive, guarded, or hostile? Is the client calm and sitting quietly or pacing and restless? Does the client appear to be attending to stimuli within his own mind (such as picking at the air or talking to empty space)? Note if the client has any motor tics or other unusual motor movements (which may be indicative of medication side effects), or if the client is using any unusual gesturing.

Mood and Affect

Mood and affect are assessed together. In general, a client's mood reflects overall emotional state. Mood is fairly consistent, whereas affect is the current emotional presentation and may be situation-dependent or change rapidly. A dysphoric mood indicates the client is persistently depressed, lethargic, apathetic, or down. It is usually accompanied by a depressed affect, but the affect may also be described as anxious or irritable. A euphoric mood is an elevated emotional state that may be associated with an affect that is giddy, cheerful, or excessively bright. A labile affect is one that is rapidly changing and unpredictable — the client may be cheerful, then suddenly becomes enraged with little provocation, or may burst into tears unexpectedly. Dysphoric moods are often associated with depression while euphoric moods may be associated with mania. Substance abuse will affect the client's mood in many ways depending on the degree of intoxication, substance used, and any withdrawal symptoms. Clients may also be described as having an affect that is flat, or blunted. Some medications can interfere with the physical expression of an emotion through blunting the emotions, or impacting negatively on the facial muscles. A client who is slow to respond emotionally, or responds at a degree less than expected, may be referred to as blunted. A client who demonstrates no emotional response at all may be considered as having a flat affect.

Thought Processes

Thought processes refer to the way thoughts are organized and structured. Normally, thoughts are logical and sequential, and easily understood by others (in the absence of a known speech or communication disorder). Clients with disorganized thoughts may seem to have nonsensical speech. They may have difficulty in performing simple activities such as bathing or eating without assistance, even in the absence of a physical impairment. The client may mix up or confuse medications when a structured system is not available (such as a weekly pill dispenser). Thoughts also may be rapid, racing, or slowed. Poverty-of-thoughts occurs when the client has a paucity of ideas or content of thoughts — questions are answered with one or two words, and the client may be unable to expand or utilize imagination. Thoughts can be abstract or concrete. In the following common proverb, *"A rolling stone gathers no moss,"* an abstract-thinking person will attempt to analyze and interpret the meaning of the statement, whereas a concrete-thinking person may answer, *"When you roll rocks, they don't get moss on them."* Tangential thoughts are seen when a client loses the central thread of a conversation. The nurse will note that one idea leads to another, which then leads to a third idea, and so forth. *"I came here in an ambulance, the driver was a man. I was married to a man once. I had a beautiful wedding. My sister makes flower arrangements for weddings. I hate my sister!"* is an example of a tangential thought process. The term flight-of-ideas may also be used to describe a client's thought processes: *"I came here in an ambulance. I wish I had more money! Did you see that TV show on Pekinese dogs the other night?"* When a client is experiencing flight-of-ideas, thoughts are somewhat random and have little association with one another. Word-salad is another phenomenon seen when assessing a client's thought processes. In a word-salad, there are no logical connections, and the thoughts are jumbled, *"I don't. Here, he said. My house. Mouse. Spouse."* The previous statement also gives an example of clang associations — or using words because they have a similar sound and not because of the actual meanings of the word. Lastly, a client may use neologisms, or words that don't exist in the English language. Words such as "frugelzip" or "rappeliciosity" will have a meaning that is clear only to the client.

Thought Content

Thought content refers to what the client is thinking about. Initially, it is helpful to assess for preoccupations or obsessions on real-life events, such as finances, employment, or relationships. An intrusive thought is an idea that comes unbidden, that occurs when the client has difficulty thinking about anything else. Ruminative thoughts are thoughts that seem to be "stuck" in the client's mind, much like a cow that will "ruminate" by chewing repeatedly. An obsessive client will tend to have ruminative thoughts that may be unusual in nature such as a desire to check the door repeatedly to ensure it is locked, or the belief that germs may be everywhere. Often, obsessive thoughts will lead to compulsive behaviors — such as ritualized handwashing — in part as an attempt to ameliorate those thoughts and their accompanying anxiety.

Two particular thought content problems are of essential importance: hallucinations and delusions. Hallucinations are disordered sensory perceptions. Auditory, visual, olfactory, gustatory, or tactile symptoms may be present. Auditory hallucinations, such as hearing voices, occur most often in the presence of a primary psychiatric illness. Visual hallucinations are most commonly seen in psychiatric disorders and in delirium states, such as those caused by alcohol withdrawal or drug toxicity (including prescription medications). Olfactory and gustatory hallucinations are rare in psychiatric illnesses, but are quite common as prodromal symptoms of an impending seizure. Occasionally a psychiatric client will report a tactile hallucination ("hands touching me," "bugs crawling on me"), but these are more often associated with alcohol or drug withdrawal states. When working with a client experiencing hallucinations, it is important to remember that the brain actually perceives the reported sensation and, to the client, it is very real. Pointing out that the hallucination does not exist is usually fruitless and may jeopardize the development of a secure nurse-client relationship.

Delusions are false beliefs. The client experiencing a delusion is certain that something is true, when there is no substantiating evidence to prove these beliefs. Paranoid delusions are common in mental health clients. Paranoid clients are usually quite frightened, as they may believe they are being watched, monitored, or spied upon by others. They may report cars following them or mysterious phone calls late at night. Occasionally a client with paranoia may fear being poisoned and refuse medications or even food. Religious delusions are another common phenomena. Clients having a religious delusion may feel persecuted by demons, or may be very excited about a special relationship with God or with angels. The health care provider needs to exert further care in obtaining a thorough history to determine a client's baseline religious beliefs so as not to label a thought as delusional when it is a well-accepted belief within the client's social network. Somatic delusions are uncomfortable beliefs that there is something terribly wrong with one's body. Some clients may believe that their bowel is necrotic or dead, or that their brain is missing. Other delusions may exist from a belief that aliens are broadcasting signals to one's loved ones have been replaced by clones. It is always essential to determine the feeling states that are produced by the client's delusional thoughts. Paranoid thoughts will drive fear and fight-or-flight responses. The client may set up protective "traps" around the home to prevent others from entering. Religious delusions may be pleasant and make the client feel special, or they may be so persecutory that the client becomes depressed and suicidal. Somatic delusions can lead to excess visits to family practitioners and emergency departments, and result in the label of "hypochondriac" for the client.

"Ideas of reference" is a thought content that occurs when the client believes that events in the environment have a personal connection to the self. Clients may report that television news broadcasters are giving them messages, or that ambulance sirens mean that something bad is about to happen. Occasionally these beliefs are so strong that the client has a great deal of discomfort with any form of media for fear of hidden meanings or messages. Sometimes ideas of reference are associated with grandiosity, or the belief that one is especially important or powerful. An elderly homemaker who suddenly believes to be the next Marilyn Monroe or Julia Roberts may be experiencing grandiosity. Grandiose clients attempt to convince others of their importance, and may present as rude or arrogant to the casual observer.

Memory and Cognition

Cognitive abilities are those elements of thinking that determine attention, concentration, perception, reasoning, intellect, and memory. They are generally thought of as "higher functioning" areas of thought. Attention span is particularly important in evaluating the mental status of children. An inability to attend to a task for an adequate length of time will impair learning. Decreased concentration levels and distractibility may be seen in clients with attentional problems, as well as clients who are depressed, or impaired due to chemical substances. Perception and reasoning can be evaluated by asking the client to perform simple multi-step tasks such as "write a sentence using your name in it" or "count backwards from 100 by 3's." An evaluation of intellectual capability is often quite detailed and lengthy, involving psychological testing. Intellect is measured in "Intellectual Quotient" or IQ scores. An IQ score below 70 is considered below normal: 55-69 indicates a mild degree of mental retardation, 40-54 a moderate degree, 25-39 a severe degree, and less than 25 is considered profound. Intellect can sometimes be estimated by asking the client about years of schooling and "special education" needs as a child, but this is unreliable due to the variability of educational and cultural environments.

An assessment of memory consists of three basic parts: immediate recall, short-term memory, and long-term memory. A simple test of recall is to give the client three items to remember, such as "apple," "car," and "house" and then 5 minutes later ask the client to state those items. Immediate recall can be quickly determined by asking what a client consumed for breakfast. Short-term memory is recall of one to several days. Questions regarding family members' names or place of residence will help to assess short-term memory. Long-term memory is recall from several days to a lifetime. Asking clients where they grew up, what their parents' names were, or where they went to school will readily provide this information. Memory assessments are important to help in differentiating a thought disorder from a dementia disorder. Clients with a primary psychiatric disturbance may be delusional in their beliefs, but extremely accurate in memory and recital of facts and dates. A client with early dementia will generally lose some short-term memory first, progressing to immediate recall, then finally to long-term memory loss. Clients with dementia may initially present with delusional beliefs as well. "Orientation" is a phrase commonly utilized in health care settings. "Oriented x 3" usually means that clients know who they are, where they are at the present time, and the approximate time, date, and day. A disoriented person may be suffering from a dementia disorder, drug or alcohol intoxication or withdrawal (including prescribed medications or drug interactions), or a number of physical health problems.

Insight and Motivation

When clients appear to have a good understanding of their illness, and steps necessary to treat or manage their disorder, then they are said to have good insight. The determination of a client's level of insight is often associated with the treatment compliance. Presumably, understanding leads to compliance. "Knowledge deficit" is a commonly used nursing diagnosis to indicate that there is a lack of understanding of either the disease process or its treatment, which can be remediated through proper education. Occasionally the nurse will encounter clients who have good insight into their illness, and have been well educated, but continues to demonstrate noncompliance with recommended treatment. This apparent lack of motivation may be related to factors other than education. The nurse should ask these clients about possible barriers to treatment such as poor finances or a lack of health insurance. The stigma of having a psychiatric diagnosis may lead the client to feel ashamed or angry. Anger may be causing the client to intentionally deny and refuse adequate treatment.

Judgment

The choices that clients make in their health care treatments are a reflection of their judgment. The diabetic client who continues to eat sugary desserts is demonstrating poor judgment, as is the alcoholic client who continues to go to nightclubs. The client, who recognizes that an increase in paranoia is a sign of decompensation and seeks out emergency treatment, is demonstrating good judgment. Judgment and insight are linked, but are not always positively correlated. Assessing and understanding a client's ability to make good or poor choices is invaluable in planning care.

Safety

Finally, an evaluation of safety is important in any mental status assessment. The essential areas to examine include safety to the self and safety to others. The nurse should determine if a client has been intentionally or unintentionally harming himself recently, or has any thoughts or urges to do so.

Clients experiencing extreme emotional pain may self-mutilate by cutting or burning their arms, legs, or trunk. Although this is not considered suicidal behavior, it is high-risk in that infection and scarring may result and the client is obviously in distress. When suicidal thoughts are noted, inpatient treatment should be considered. Assessing suicide risk consists of asking the client about means to harm oneself, and the availability of those means. A hunter who thinks about shooting himself is at much higher risk than the office worker who doesn't own a gun. Determining the lethality of the means available is also essential. Overdosing on prescription cardiac agents or tricyclic antidepressants is far more dangerous than overdosing on selective serotonin reuptake inhibitors. Many adolescent clients cause serious liver damage every year by overdosing on relatively small amounts of acetaminophen, which is easily accessible to a minor. Another important assessment tool is to determine if the client has developed a suicide plan. A well-developed suicide plan with means at hand may necessitate forcing an involuntary hospital stay, whereas an impulsive episode of self-mutilat-

ing may be best treated by an intensive outpatient program and family supervision.

The nurse should also determine the degree of risk to others involved. There are two distinct areas in which psychiatric clients lose their rights to confidentiality: a direct threat to harm or kill another person, and the report of child abuse, neglect, or molestation. "Duty to warn" is the term that refers to the duty carried by the health care provider to notify another individual when a threat has been made against that individual's life. The nurse must use all means necessary to reasonably contact the individual including notifying the police. In most health care settings, there are policies to be followed to ensure the report is made accurately and documented appropriately. If a client tells the nurse about the knowledge of the abuse, molestation, or neglect of a minor child, then the nurse is obligated to report this to the local child protective services. Not reporting suspected abuse or neglect constitutes a major ethical problem, and may jeopardize the nurse's license and employment. Again, most health care facilities have policies in place to coordinate these types of reports. Ultimately, the nurse is responsible for seeing that the report has been made.

NURSING CARE PLAN

Sally is a 25-year-old single woman with a history of numerous psychiatric inpatient stays with the diagnosis of bipolar disorder. The nurse is interviewing her in a hospital room where she was admitted for an acute manic episode. The following dialogue between the nurse and the client will be utilized to demonstrate the application of the nursing process in writing a nursing care plan:

Nurse: *"I understand you've been having some trouble sleeping?"*

Sally: *"I haven't slept in 3 or 4 days. But I don't need sleep! Don't you see? I have been rebirthed in the spirit of our lady, Athena, the goddess of light and dark. She has given me the ability to see far-reaching into the future! Would you like me to tell you about your true love? Love is grand. Love is dandy. Love is like candy. Sandy beaches and moonlight. True light. Blue light is shining on me. There! Do you see!?"*

Nurse: *"Let's focus on what we can do to help you get some rest. When this happened to you last fall, you were able to get some relief with sleeping medication."*

Sally: *"Medicine. Schmedicine. I don't need any of that drug stuff. The stars will take me away sailing away and I'll never sleep again. (Starts to cry.) Oh, can't I ever be like everyone else? Why does this keep happening? If only I could get some rest."*

Nurse: *"Remember when you were here before. It only lasted a little while, then you got better. And you will get better again. The first step is to get you settled down. Later, I'm going to get you a cup of warm milk and some extra blankets. Then I'll set up the relaxation tape we keep here in the foyer outside your room. I'll give you a sleeping pill and play the relaxation tape. I'll bet you'll drift right off and feel much better tomorrow."*

Sally: *"I don't know if it will help...but...okay. I'll try anything. You'll be here won't you? To make sure I'm okay? I'm always scared in the hospital."*

Nurse: *"I work until 11:30 p.m. I'll check on you before I go home."*

Problem Listing

- Inadequate
- Labile moods
- Mild grandiosity
- Anxiety over being in the hospital
- Potential for medication noncompliance

Primary Nursing Diagnosis

Sleep disturbance (insomnia) due to the acute exacerbation of a manic episode as demonstrated by 3 nights with no sleep and a labile mood.

Long-term Treatment Goal

Client will sleep every night for a minimum of 6 hours for 5 days in a row prior to discharge.

Short-term Objectives

1. Client will verbalize the importance of getting a good night's sleep.

2. Client will ask for the as needed (p.r.n.) medications that are available.

Interventions

1. Staff will administer a bedtime (h.s.) sedative at 10:00 p.m. and document results.

2. Staff will offer warm milk and extra blankets at h.s.

3. Staff will turn down lights and keep noise to a minimum.

4. Staff will teach the client deep breathing techniques utilizing relaxation cassette tape or soft music.

5. Staff will utilize a nonconfrontational, supportive approach with the client to support a sense of security and safety.

The final stage of the nursing process, evaluating the effectiveness of interventions and the completion of objectives, is done on a daily basis. In the example given above, the client slept 4 hours only. The nurse documented the objectives as partially met and continued the care plan with no alterations.

EXAM QUESTIONS

CHAPTER 3
Questions 16-22

16. A nursing action conducive to obtaining a thorough and accurate nursing history would be

    a. keeping the TV and radio turned off, and distraction to a minimum.

    b. obtaining information only from secondary sources and records.

    c. interviewing the client at the nurse's station for safety.

    d. focusing only on psychiatric symptomatology.

17. Bobby is a 46-year-old man with schizophrenia. On interviewing him, you note the following statement, *"I came in to get my meds adjusted. I take meds for a lot of things. I get my meds at the grocery store. I haven't gotten any groceries yet this week. Next week I am planning a trip to France. Do you like the French? I bought some French's mustard."* This is an example of

    a. paranoid thoughts.

    b. disorientation to person-place-time.

    c. drug intoxication.

    d. tangential thoughts.

18. Sam is a 19-year-old client who presents with the following statement, *"I had to come in here! There was a man stalking me outside of my apartment. I stayed up all night watching and I kept seeing shadows. I'm sure the government is in on it! Can you help me to prove there's a conspiracy against me?"* This statement represents

    a. religious preoccupations.

    b. flight-of-ideas.

    c. paranoid delusions.

    d. auditory hallucinations.

19. When evaluating safety in a mental status assessment, the statement that best reflects a high risk for a suicide attempt is

    a. *"Next week my kids are coming to visit and I am so stressed that I want to just escape from it all."*

    b. *"I don't see a future for myself. I've been thinking a lot lately about dying and how peaceful it would be to take my heart pills and go to sleep forever."*

    c. *"I wish I had a knife! I get so tensed up that I just want to stab something!"*

    d. *"Everyone hates me. My parents and my friends think I'm dumb. I just wish I were dead!"*

20. The nurse has identified four problems that a client is experiencing. Using skills of prioritizing, the problem that should be addressed initially in the nursing care plan is

    a. sleeps less than 8 hours per night.

    b. hasn't eaten for 4 days.

    c. lacks confidence in abilities.

    d. homelessness.

21. Jack is a 45-year-old man who presents in the emergency department confused and staggering. He has had numerous past admissions for alcohol detoxification complicated by withdrawal seizures and liver failure. The nursing diagnosis most appropriate for his first 24 hours of care is

    a. ineffective denial related to guilt as evidenced by refusing to accept treatment voluntarily.

    b. ineffective family coping related to destructive family patterns as evidenced by inappropriate anger demonstrations.

    c. risk for injury related to changes in mental status and a history of seizures as evidenced by confusion and a staggering gait.

    d. impaired social interactions related to emotional lability as evidenced by tearfulness and isolation on admission.

22. Both long-term and short-term goals are best expressed in measurable behaviors. The most appropriately worded objective in the following examples is:

    a. Client will understand how to use a Nicoderm® patch prior to discharge.

    b. Client will know how to use a Nicoderm® patch prior to discharge.

    c. Client will demonstrate how to apply a Nicoderm® patch prior to discharge.

    d. Client will comply with his Nicoderm® patch treatment prior to discharge.

CHAPTER 4

SCHIZOPHRENIA AND RELATED DISORDERS

CHAPTER OBJECTIVE

At the end of this chapter the reader will be able to identify symptoms of a thought disorder and discuss appropriate nursing care and medication treatment.

LEARNING OBJECTIVES

At the end of this chapter, the reader will be able to

1. describe the symptoms of schizophrenia.

2. differentiate schizophrenia from other psychotic disorders.

3. discuss antipsychotic medications and their side effects.

SCHIZOPHRENIA: ETIOLOGY AND DEVELOPMENT

Schizophrenia is a severe psychiatric disorder that is chronic and may be very disabling to the individual. The incidence of schizophrenia in the population is about 1% with morbidity approximately the same for men and women. The average age of onset varies slightly with the majority of men becoming ill either at around ages 20-25, or around ages 30-35. Women tend to experience a disease onset average approximately 5 years later

than men. After age 45, the ratio of women to men in newly diagnosed cases becomes 2 to 1. Schizophrenia is believed to be a brain-based medical disorder with distinct, yet unknown, neurobiological causes. Although schizophrenia has been noted to have familial tendencies (first-degree relatives have a risk for the disorder at a rate of 10 times the general population), more than 60% of persons with schizophrenia have no family history of the disorder and the concordance rate for monozygotic (identical) twins is only 50%. This would imply that nongenetic factors are also important in the development of the disease (Nasrallah & Smeltzer, 2002).

To diagnose schizophrenia, there must be an occurrence of symptoms that lasts for 6 months and include at least 1 month of clear positive or negative symptom groups (*DSM-IV-TR*, 2002). Positive symptoms may include hallucinations of any type, delusional beliefs, grossly disorganized behavior or speech, or catatonic behaviors. Negative symptoms are more difficult to identify and reflect a loss of normal functioning. Three major negative symptom characteristics are associated with most clients with schizophrenia. These include affective flattening, alogia, and avolition. Affective flattening refers to an apparent lack of emotional responsivity in the client. The client may demonstrate poor eye contact, few facial gestures, and reduced body contact. The client may be able to briefly smile or laugh, but both the intensity and the duration of the emotional response are impaired. Alogia, also referred to as a poverty-of-speech, is exhibited by brief replies to questions and a lack of elaboration or colorful details in speech content. The client may answer questions with only one or two words then lapse into silence. Alogia is associated with a diminished range and content of thoughts, reflected in the decrease in speech. Lastly, avolition is exhibited by a decreased ability to initiate or maintain activities. Clients may appear to be staring off into space for long periods of time, and may require frequent reminders to participate in daily activities. Together, negative symptoms have a profound impact on social relationships, employment, continued education, self-care abilities, and other life endeavors. Medication treatment of schizophrenia consists of antipsychotic agents.

To diagnose schizophrenia, six criterion are provided by the *DSM-IV-TR.*

1. *Characteristic symptoms:* Two or more of the following must be present, each for most of a 1-month period:
    a. delusions
    b. hallucinations
    c. disorganized speech
    d. grossly disorganized or catatonic behavior
    e. negative symptoms (affective flattening, alogia, or avolition)

2. *Social/occupational dysfunction:* one or more major areas of functioning (work, relationships), or self-care are markedly below the level expected for the individual (child), or the level achieved previously (adult).

3. *Duration:* Continuous symptoms persist for at least 6 months with at least 1 month of criterion-1 symptoms.

4. *Schizoaffective and Mood Disorder exclusion:* No major depressive, manic, or mixed mood episodes have occurred concurrently with the criterion-1 symptoms (or mood symptoms are brief).

5. *Substance/general medical condition exclusion:* Drugs, alcohol, or medical conditions cannot be associated with the symptoms.

6. *Relationship to a pervasive developmental disorder:* In the presence of a history of autism or pervasive developmental disorder, prominent symptoms of delusions or hallucinations must be present for at least a month.

Schizophrenia is further differentiated in the *DSM-IV-TR* into five subtypes: paranoid, disorganized, catatonic, undifferentiated, and residual. Each of these subtypes is identified based on the symptom clusters that are experienced by the client.

Paranoid schizophrenia is expressed by an overall good organization of thought processes accompanied by delusions that may be persecutory, grandiose, jealous, religious, or even somatic. Delusions usually center on a specific theme and may be very intricate and detailed. Hallucinations may also be present. Associated mood states may be fear, anger, suspiciousness, irritability, mistrust, anxiety, arrogance, or aloofness. The combination of persecutory delusions with anger may predispose the client to violence or suicidal tendencies. There is little cognitive impairment and clients, though resistant to treatment, may respond well to antipsychotic agents. Occupational functioning and self-care abilities are impacted less with this subtype than with the other four.

Clients with disorganized schizophrenia have a much greater difficulty in managing their affairs and living independently. Speech, thoughts, and behavior may all be disorganized and the client may demonstrate a flat or inappropriate affect. Hallucinations and delusions, when present, may be scattered and aren't as clearly thematic in nature as in paranoid schizophrenia. Clients who are acutely ill may be unable to complete a sentence, express a simple idea, or perform basic self-care activities, such as bathing and dressing. Associated features may include odd or bizarre grimacing or behavioral mannerisms.

The essential feature of catatonic schizophrenia is an extreme psychomotor slowing or retardation that may cause stupor, immobility, mutism, echolalia (echoing others' words or phrases), echopraxia (imitating the behavior of others), negativism, or even agitated activity that is non-goal oriented and purposeless. Catalepsy (also called "waxy flexibility") is an unusual symptom that may allow the health care provider to "pose" an immobile client, much like a department store manikin, and the client will hold his position for a long period of time. During an acute phase, the client will need a great deal of nursing care to prevent self-harm, malnutrition, dehydration, or injury. Hallucinations are difficult to assess, and the client may seem to be devoid of emotions or affect.

A client with undifferentiated schizophrenia has symptoms that meet the criterion-1 category, but do not meet the criteria to be classified as paranoid, disorganized, or catatonic. Occasionally this diagnosis is used when the clinical picture is quite variable.

Residual schizophrenia is diagnosed when a client has had at least one episode of the disorder, but the current presentation is without significant positive symptoms. Associated positive symptoms may be present (odd mannerisms or gesturing), and there is continued evidence of negative symptoms. Any delusions or hallucinations are minimal, and there is not an associated change in affect. Residual type schizophrenia may be brief and occur between acute episodes, or it may become a long-term, "baseline" presentation.

SCHIZOAFFECTIVE DISORDER

Schizoaffective disorder is a neurobiological (brain-based) disorder in which there is a clear episode of clinical depression, mania, or mixed depressive and manic symptoms concurrent with criterion-1 symptoms of schizophrenia. The symptoms cannot be due to the effect of substances (e.g., amphetamines), or a medical condition. The mood symptoms must be present for a "prominent period of time." This time period requires clinical judgment, but can be no less than 1 full week in the case of mania or mixed mania/depression, or 2 weeks in the case of depression. Prominent hallucinations or delusions must also be present during the course of the illness (which differentiates this disorder from a primary major depression or bipolar illness). Two subtypes of schizoaffective disorder are identified: bipolar type and depressed type. Medication treatment of a schizoaffective disorder may include antipsychotics, antidepressants, and/or mood stabilizers.

OTHER PSYCHOTIC DISORDERS

Other, less common, disorders related to thought processes and thought content are presented in the *DSM-IV-TR*. A brief description of each follows.

1. Schizophreniform disorder — the client meets the first three criteria for schizophrenia, but the duration of the disorder is less than 6 months. Impaired social or occupational functioning is not required.

2. Delusional disorder — the client has one or more irrational or inaccurate belief that persists for at least 1 month. There may be hallucinations associated with the delusion. Behavior and psychosocial functioning are not impaired. Several subtypes exist: erotomanic (the belief that another person is in love with the individual), grandiose (the belief that one has a great, but unrecognized, talent, insight, or discovery, or that one has a special relationship with someone famous), jealous (the belief that a spouse or

lover is unfaithful), persecutory (the belief that one is being conspired against), somatic (the belief that something is gravely wrong with one's body), mixed (seen when no one theme emerges), or unspecified (when the delusional belief cannot be readily determined).

3. Brief psychotic disorder — sudden onset of at least one of the criterion-1 symptoms with no known etiology (e.g., substances or illness) lasting from 1 day to 1 month with full return to a premorbid state. May be seen after a traumatic psychosocial stressor occurs.

4. Shared psychotic disorder — formerly called folie à deux, a delusion develops in an individual who is closely involved with another person who already is experiencing a psychotic disorder with prominent delusions.

5. Psychotic disorder due to a general medical condition — diagnosed when an individual develops criterion-1 symptoms that can be clearly linked to a medical event, such as a head injury, dementia, or a metabolic disturbance.

6. Substance-induced psychotic disorder — diagnosed when the individual develops criterion-1 symptoms that are associated with either the use or the withdrawal of a substance such as alcohol, illegal drugs, prescription medications, or a variety of other offending agents.

7. Psychotic disorder not otherwise specified — used when the etiology of the psychosis is unclear, or a full diagnostic workup has not yet been completed (inadequate information).

ANTIPSYCHOTIC MEDICATIONS

Medications have been used in psychiatric disorders since they were first available. Early mental health treatment consisted primarily of chemical restraints on behaviors. Various concoctions were used — all containing blends of opiates,

alcohol, or other sedating chemicals. The first generation of medications specifically targeted to reduce the symptoms of schizophrenia was developed in the early 1950s with chlorpromazine (Thorazine®), a phenothiazine agent with pronounced antihistamine properties. Several others soon followed including trifluoperazine (Stelazine®) and thioridazine (Mellaril®). Between 1952 and 1975, laboratories worked to alter the phenothiazine compound to develop several different classes of antipsychotic medications, with more than 10 first-generation agents (Nasrallah & Smeltzer, 2002). Although efficacious for the positive symptoms of schizophrenia and psychotic disorders, the traditional agents are all high in side effects and do little to ameliorate the negative symptoms. Table 4-1 presents an overview of the traditional antipsychotic agents developed along with a comparison of their potency levels and side effect profiles.

The primary mechanism of action of the traditional antipsychotic agents is postsynaptic dopamine receptor antagonism — that is, the medication binds with the dopamine receptors in the neurons of the brain, thus reducing (or blocking) the transmission of the neurotransmitter dopamine through the brain. Dopamine blockade of these agents is nonspecific, which has contributed to numerous unwanted neurological effects, the worst of these being a medication-induced pseudoparkinsonism secondary to dopamine blockade in the extrapyramidal tract of the brain (commonly referred to as extrapyramidal syndrome) and tardive dyskinesia whose etiology is unclear. Symptoms of extrapyramidal syndrome include tremors of the skeletal muscles (most commonly noticed in the upper extremities), a blunting or stiffening of the facial muscles resulting in a mask-like facial expression, slowed gait (bradykinesia), shuffling gait, stiffening of the skeletal muscles, a purposeless sense of restlessness, and occasionally a sudden muscle dystonia, or unremitting contrac-

TABLE 4-1: TRADITIONAL ANTIPSYCHOTIC MEDICATIONS IN COMMON USAGE

Generic Name	Trade Name	Relative Potency	EPS Risk	TD Risk	Ortho B/P Risk	Sedation	Weight Gain	Anticholinergic Properties	Comments
Chlorpromazine	Thorazine®	+	++	++	+++	++	+++	+++	1st antipsychotic developed
Thioridazine	Mellaril®	+	+	+	+++	+++	+++	+++	Q-Tc prolongation problematic
Fluphenazine	Prolixin®	+++	+++	+++	+	+	+	++	Available in long-acting decanoate injection
Perphenazine	Trilafon®	++	++	++	+++	++	+	++	Available combined w/amitriptyline (Triavil®)
Trifluoperazine	Stelazine®	+++	+++	+++	++	+	+	++	
Thiothixene	Navane®	+++	+++	+++	+	++	++	++	
Haloperidol	Haldol®	+++	+++	++	+	+	++	++	Available in long-acting decanoate injection
Loxapine	Loxitane®	++	++	++	++	++	+	+	
Molindone	Moban®	++	++	++	+	+	+	+	
Pimozide	Orap®	+++	+++	++	++	++	+	+++	Q-Tc prolongation a concern. Primary use is in Tourette's syndrome.

+++ High
++ Moderate
+ Low

tion, often noted in the muscles of the neck, shoulders, or eyes. Extrapyramidal syndrome symptoms often may be partially or completely relieved by the addition of anticholinergic medications (see Table 4-2). Tardive dyskinesia is a central nervous system (CNS) disorder more likely to occur after prolonged exposure to traditional antipsychotics. Tardive dyskinesia is characterized by abnormal, choreiform movements of the muscles resulting is repetitive, often slow or writhing, body movements. Tardive dyskinesia does not respond to anti-

cholinergic medications and it rarely remits spontaneously. There is no current treatment for tardive dyskinesia, although switching to one of the newer antipsychotic agents may be useful. Some recent research has suggested that antioxidants, such as vitamin E, may reduce some of the symptoms. When utilized, vitamin E should be administrated at 800-1,200 international units daily.

Other CNS side effects may include an elevation in prolactin levels in the brain, resulting in dysmenorrhea, reduced libido, breast enlargement, or

TABLE 4-2: MEDICATIONS USED TO TREAT EXTRAPYRAMIDAL SYNDROME EFFECTS ASSOCIATED WITH ANTIPSYCHOTICS

Generic Name	Trade Name	Classification	Comments
Benztropine	Cogentin®	Anticholinergic	Available in PO or IM formulation
Trihexyphenidyl	Artane®	Anticholinergic	Some clients report less dry mouth
Amantadine	Symmetrel®	Dopamine agonist	Antiviral activities as well as EPS tx.
Bromocriptine	Parlodel®	Dopamine agonist	Inhibits prolactin release
Diphenhydramine	Benadryl®	Antihistamine	Often used in child/adolescents
Propanolol	Inderal®	Beta-blocker	Primarily for tremors
Lorazepam	Ativan®	Benzodiazepine	Useful for restlessness, pacing

false breast milk (galactorrhea); inappropriate antidiuretic hormone resulting in water toxicity (also called polygenic polydipsia); seizures (rarely); thermoregulatory abnormalities resulting in hyperthermia or hypothermia; and neuroleptic malignant syndrome which is a poorly understood syndrome where body temperature rises rapidly and skeletal muscle breakdown occurs. Without emergency treatment, neuroleptic malignant syndrome can be life threatening.

Non-CNS side effects are also prominent with traditional antipsychotics. Antihistamine-like properties cause drowsiness and an increased appetite (and weight gain). Cardiovascular effects may occur and are evidenced by orthostatic hypotension, tachycardia (rapid heart beat), and prolongation of the Q-Tc interval in electrical conduction through the heart, which may trigger a sudden cardiac arrest associated with a ventricular fibrillation known as torsades de pointes. Thioridazine (Mellaril®) now carries a black-box warning due to it's potential for Q-Tc prolongation. Anticholinergic properties of traditional antipsychotics can cause dry mouth, constipation, and urinary retention. Some blood dyscrasias may occur with traditional antipsychotics. Altered glucose metabolism and an increased risk for diabetes are seen in clients taking antipsychotic agents. Usually this is an adult-onset, type II diabetes associated with obesity, but there have been reports of diabetic ketoacidosis in the absence of significant weight gain along with an increase in serum lipid levels and triglycerides. Ocular disorders have emerged in clients taking traditional antipsychotics: an increase in retinal pigmentation can be seen as well as an increase in cataract development. Agents used to treat extrapyramidal syndrome may also cause ocular disturbances — primarily blurred vision, dry eyes, and acute glaucoma symptoms. Gastrointestinal problems include dry mouth, constipation, elevated liver enzymes, and even paralytic ileus. Finally,

photosensitivity reactions may occur causing excess sunburn and rashes (Nasrallah & Smeltzer, 2002).

Special consideration must be made with utilizing antipsychotic agents during pregnancy. There is no current evidence of teratogenicity (congenital abnormalities or birth defects), but the literature is sparse. A risk/benefit analysis should be done that considers the potential benefit to the expectant mother in terms of psychiatric stability, and prenatal care, and compares that to the risk of decompensated mental illness including postpartum psychosis and danger to the infant. Breast-feeding is often discouraged due to the lack of information on the effects on the infant.

Certain ethnic populations may metabolize antipsychotic agents differently or at a slower rate than in the general population. African American and Asian populations tend to have a genetic variant of the enzyme CYP2D6 — resulting in slower drug metabolism and a higher incidence of extrapyramidal syndrome and tardive dyskinesia. Lower drug dosages may be indicated.

Tobacco induces cytochrome enzymes and can significantly increase the oxidation of some antipsychotics, reducing the serum concentrations and bioavailability of the drug. When a client chooses to stop smoking, serum medication levels may rise and cause an increase in side effects at the same dosage as previously taken.

New Generation Antipsychotics

After four decades, it quickly became evident that newer medications were needed. Drug development started to focus on continued treatment efficacy but additionally targeting the negative symptoms of avolition, alogia, and affective flattening, as well as attempting to reduce the noxious side effects of the traditional agents. The first of these newer agents was clozapine (Clozaril®). Clozapine was initially discovered in 1959; however, the trends in medicating at the time dictated that psychotic remission was synonymous with extrapyramidal syndrome emergence. As clozapine had no extrapyramidal syndrome side effects, it was initially thought to be a poor medication. Research continued and it was launched in Europe in 1972. The United States did not initially approve clozapine because of concerns about hypotension and increased seizure risk. Three years after its European launch, it became clear that there were several cases of agranulocytosis leading to death. It was removed from the market at that time. Clozapine continued to be studied, and it was reintroduced to the U.S. Food and Drug Administration (FDA) for approval in the 1980s, due to its marked superiority in treatment efficacy over traditional agents. In 1988, the FDA approved clozapine only after other medications had been tried and failed, and with the caveat that all clients receiving the drug would have to have weekly white blood cell (WBC) count monitoring. A few years ago, this restriction was eased to allow clients who have been receiving clozapine on a regular basis for over 6 months to get WBC counts done every 2 weeks. Even without extrapyramidal syndrome or tardive dyskinesia side effects, clozapine can cause hypotension, sialorrhea (excess salivation), sedation, weight gain (and increased risk for diabetes), and increased seizure risk. Additionally, the drug is metabolized quickly in the body and a client will rapidly decompensate after only a few missed doses. Rebound hypertension and tachycardia may occur with sudden withdrawal of clozapine.

After clozapine, several other new generation, "atypical" antipsychotics were introduced. These include risperidone (Risperdal®) in 1994, olanzapine (Zyprexa®) in 1996, quetiapine (Seroquel®) in 1997, ziprasidone (Geodon®) in 2001, and aripiprazole (Abilify™) in 2002. A distinguishing characteristic of the newer generation drugs is that, although they are still primarily dopamine antagonist, they also have serotonin reuptake blocking effects, which seem to be associated with an improvement in the negative symptoms including cognitive functioning of schizophrenia and other chronic, psychotic disorders. (See Table 4-3.) Olanzapine (Zyprexa®) is also approved for use as a primary agent in bipolar mood disorders.

TABLE 4-3: NEW GENERATION ANTIPSYCHOTIC MEDICATIONS

Generic Name	Trade Name	EPS Risk	TD Risk	Ortho B/P	Sedation Risk	Weight Gain	Anticholinergic Properties	Comments
Clozapine	Clozaril®	+	+	+++	+++	+++	+	• WBC monitoring required due to risk of agranulocytosis • Increased seizure risk
Risperdone	Risperdal®	++	+	+	++	++	++	• Pronounced prolactin elevation in some clients • Frequent pediatric usage
Olanzapine	Zyprexa® Zidis®	+	+	+	+++	+++	+	• Weight gain associated with type II diabetes • Zidis® is rapid-dissolving wafer formulation
Quetiapine	Seroquel®	+	+	++	++	++	+	• Pronounced antianxiety effects • Increase in pediatric usage
Ziprasidone	Geodon®	+	+	+	+	+	+	• Contraindicated in cardiac disease over Q-Tc prolongation concerns
Aripiprazole	Abilify™	+	+	+	+	+	+	• New product. Released November 2002.

+++	High
++	Moderate
+	Low

NURSING CARE OF THE CLIENT WITH SCHIZOPHRENIA AND RELATED DISORDERS

Psychiatric nursing roles center around the following areas of holistic care: maintaining safety of the client and staff; assessing for mental and physical health alterations; supporting basic needs for nutrition, hydration, sleep, warmth, elimination, hygiene; and supporting and educating the client, family, and significant others about the disease process and appropriate treatments, which may include medications.

Safety and risk assessment involve monitoring of clients for any evidence of harmful behavior to self, or any signs in increasing tension or agitation. Most health care facilities provide training for staff in crisis prevention, or how to de-escalate a situation. In an outpatient setting, the nurse should watch for clues that a client is becoming increasingly psychotic, manic, or depressed. Changes in mental status can be associated with emergent suicidal or violent thoughts, or severe disorganization leading to an inability to provide basic self-care. Medication changes or even hospitalization (voluntary or involuntary) may be necessary. Clients who are abusing alcohol or drugs in combination with an underlying psychiatric disorder are at particular risk for self-injury or harm to others.

Seclusion is the involuntary confinement of a client to a room where the door is locked or the client is otherwise unable to leave. Restraint is defined as any method of physically restricting a client's freedom of movement in any way (Keltner, Schwecke, & Bostrom, 2003). Secluding and/or restraining mentally ill persons has been used for hundreds of years. Today, the client must be presenting a clear and imminent danger to oneself or others in order to justify the use of seclusion or restraints. It is inappropriate to seclude or restrain a client for the purposes of punishment. The nurse must chart the justification for the seclusion and restraints, the type of restraint used, alternative means that were tried before resorting to seclusion and restraints, the amount of time the client was in seclusion or restraints, the objective(s) to be reached by utilizing seclusion and restraints, regular safety checks of the client, and the measures taken to ensure hydration, nutrition, and proper toileting for the client while in seclusion or restraints. As needed, or p.r.n., orders are never deemed to be appropriate. Each occurrence is treated as a separate and distinct event and must be documented as such. Seclusion and restraints is not appropriate for outpatient or residential settings caring for clients with psychiatric disorders. In many hospitals, physicians are required to assess the client within 30-60 minutes of the application of seclusion and restraints.

Administering medications, teaching about the effects and side effects of those medications, assessing for medication efficacy and monitoring for noncompliance are important nursing interventions. Antipsychotic medications come in oral and injectable intramuscular (IM) formulations. The nurse should document the medication given as well as any observations of the client during that time, paying particular attention to CNS side effects such as extrapyramidal syndrome and tardive dyskinesia. For p.r.n. medications, the effectiveness and outcome should also be noted.

The psychiatric nurse fulfills a vital role in performing both mental and physical health assessments. Generalized knowledge of body systems and disease processes is essential. The nurse is often viewed as a resource by non-nursing and non-medical counseling and support staff. Identifying symptoms and placing symptom clusters into a framework will help the nurse in learning to differentiate an acute psychiatric disturbance from a medical disease (i.e., presenting symptoms of anxiety and paranoid delusions may be triggered by a decreased oxygen level secondary to congestive heart failure). The ability to prioritize and triage in emergency situations is essential.

Supporting clients in nutrition, hydration, elimination, hygiene, and other basic needs is especially important in the acute phase of a psychiatric decompensation. Clients who are disorganized or catatonic may suffer from fluid and electrolyte imbalances. Constipation can lead to intense discomfort and bowel perforations necessitating surgery. Poor hygiene can result in skin lesions or parasites (head lice) as well as social ostracization. Inadequate dental care may lead to cavities or infections of the mouth, jaw, and oral structures. Occasionally, a mouth infection becomes systemic and can cause septic shock. Assisting clients with basic care will help them preserve their dignity and integrity.

Education is a cornerstone of psychiatric nursing. Individuals with mental disorders are not "sick" in the traditional sense of the word; rather they are experiencing an acute disruption in role performance and overall functioning. Assisting the client and family members or significant others in understanding psychiatric illnesses and their treatment will promote better treatment compliance and improve overall health. Teaching practical skills such as relaxation techniques will provide clients with alternative coping strategies in times of increased stress. Learning to understand and recognize signs of decompensation, then to seek out help early, will decrease the length and intensity of acute illness episodes. Families with acutely ill loved ones often have difficulty in comprehending issues of personal freedom and the right to refuse treatment. The nurse can educate them about the legal process, and support them when they are feeling helpless to intervene.

SCHIZOPHRENIA CASE STUDY

Jim is a 46-year-old man diagnosed with schizophrenia, paranoid type. He first became ill at age 19 when he came home from his freshman year of college to tell his parents that CIA agents had attempted to make contact with him using the computer lab in his dormitory. He has been hospitalized six times since, with one state hospitalization lasting 18 months after he assaulted his therapist (he accused the therapist of planting listening devices in his apartment). Jim has been put on the decanoate injectable form of the antipsychotic haloperidol (Haldol®), which he receives once a month at the mental health center. The nurse notes that Jim is rocking back and forth, rubbing his fingertips together, blinking rapidly, and smacking his lips. He is also taking the anticholinergic medication benztropine (Cogentin®) to control his tremors.

He weighs 278 lb at a height of 5'11". His blood pressure is 168/110, with a heart rate of 96, and a respiratory rate of 24. Jim tells the nurse that he drinks two pots of coffee a day, and smokes two to three packs of cigarettes. He is complaining about difficulty going to sleep before 4:00 a.m. — then he is unable to waken until 1:00 p.m. the following day. Jim also reports ongoing auditory hallucinations that are derogatory in nature. The "voices" tell him, "You are worthless. They're coming to get you! They'll lock you up again! Watch out!"

NURSING CARE PLAN

Problem Listing

- Poor nutrition — overweight
- Elevated blood pressure
- Shortness of breath
- Sleep cycle disturbance
- Caffeine abuse/dependence
- Nicotine dependence

- Auditory hallucinations
- Probable tardive dyskinesia
- Threats to self-esteem due to derogatory hallucinations

Nursing Diagnoses

1. Imbalanced nutrition: more than body requirements related to excessive intake of food as evidenced by weight of 278 lb at 5'11".

2. Ineffective health maintenance related to knowledge deficit as evidenced by blood pressure reading of 168/110.

3. Sleep pattern disorder related to excess intake of caffeine late at night as evidenced by a pattern of sleeping 4:00 a.m.-1:00 p.m.

4. Disturbed sensory perceptions: auditory hallucinations related to disease process as evidenced by patient report of "hearing voices."

5. Impaired physical mobility related to antipsychotic medication treatment as evidenced by symptoms of tardive dyskinesia.

Long-term Goal

Client will have improved physical and mental health status with a decreased risk for cardiac or respiratory disease.

Short-term Objectives

1. Client will reach a goal weight of 200 lb by the end of 6 months.

2. Client will demonstrate BP readings consistently less than 140/90.

3. Client will go to sleep by 11:00 p.m. nightly.

4. Client will report decreased or eliminated auditory hallucinations.

5. Client will decrease caffeine and nicotine use by 50% in 6 months.

6. Client will verbalize the importance of regular physical activity in improving mobility.

Nursing Interventions

1. a. Educate the client about the importance of good nutrition for health.

   b. Facilitate a dietitian consult.

   c. Assist the client in identifying ways to build activity into the daily routine.

   d. Weigh the client weekly to monthly to assess progress.

2. a. Check BP with each monthly injection.

   b. Facilitate a medical exam with a family care provider to determine if an antihypertensive agent is needed.

3. a. Educate the client about the relationship between caffeine and insomnia.

   b. Teach the client relaxation techniques to utilize at bedtime.

   c. Encourage the client to set alarm clock for 8:00 a.m. daily and to get up.

   d. Advise the client to not take naps.

   e. Teach the client that cigarettes will keep him awake (not to smoke after 10:00 p.m.).

4. a. Discuss using as needed (p.r.n.) medications with the client.

   b. Educate the client about using techniques to distract himself from the hallucinations (such as listening to music).

5. a. Assist the client in setting up a schedule to decrease caffeine and nicotine use.

   b. Suggest that the client use half-caffeinated and half-decaffeinated coffee.

6. a. Assist the client in incorporating activity into a daily schedule and teach gentle stretching techniques.

EXAM QUESTIONS

CHAPTER 4
Questions 23-29

23. An example of what is meant by "positive symptoms" is

    a. good interpersonal skills and a bright, cheerful affect.

    b. hallucinations and delusions.

    c. poor eye contact and decreased thought content.

    d. rapid response to antipsychotic medication intervention.

24. Negative symptoms include

    a. grandiosity, ideas of reference, and hallucinations.

    b. depressed mood, anhedonia, and nihilism.

    c. somatic delusions, poor hygiene, and disorganization.

    d. affective flattening, alogia, and avolition.

25. A somatic delusion is a belief that

    a. your spouse is having multiple affairs.

    b. aliens are returning to earth to take you home.

    c. the IRS is plotting a conspiracy against you.

    d. something is gravely wrong with a part of your body.

26. *Terri presents in the emergency department with agitation and pressured speech. She looks to be about 30 years old, and she is very thin and emaciated. She is pacing rapidly and talks illogically of insects that are crawling in her mouth and ears and taking over her brain. Her urine drug screen comes back as positive for cocaine and cannabinoids.*

    The most likely diagnosis for this client is

    a. Schizophrenia, disorganized type.

    b. Schizoaffective disorder.

    c. Brief psychotic disorder.

    d. Substance-induced psychotic disorder.

27. The neurotransmitter that is associated both with treatment efficacy of traditional antipsychotics, as well as with extrapyramidal syndrome effects, is

    a. acetylcholine.

    b. dopamine.

    c. serotonin.

    d. gamma-amino butyric acid.

28. Doses of antipsychotics in the Asian American population as compared to the general population may need to be adjusted

    a. higher.

    b. very little.

    c. lower.

    d. by doubling.

29. In general, new generation antipsychotics have activity on

    a. dopamine and acetylcholine.

    b. dopamine and serotonin.

    c. serotonin and norepinephrine.

    d. norepinephrine and gamma-amino butyric acid.

CHAPTER 5

DEMENTIA AND DELIRIUM

CHAPTER OBJECTIVE

At the end of this chapter, the reader will be able to recognize the symptoms of a dementia disorder, differentiate it from delirium, and identify appropriate nursing measures for promoting safety and maximizing functioning.

LEARNING OBJECTIVES

At the end of this chapter, the reader will be able to

1. identify symptoms of a dementia disorder.

2. differentiate symptoms of dementia from delirium.

3. describe nursing interventions for the client with either a dementia disorder or delirium.

DEMENTIA DISORDERS: ETIOLOGY AND DEVELOPMENT

Dementia refers to the loss of thinking abilities, particularly memory, in combination with disturbances in executive functioning (the ability to think abstractly and to plan and initiate behaviors), aphasia, apraxia, or agnosia. Aphasia refers to deterioration in language functioning. Apraxia is defined as "an impaired ability to execute motor activities despite intact motor abilities, sensory function, and comprehension of the required task" (*DSM-IV-TR*, 2002). A failure to recognize or identify common objects is known as agnosia. Dementia may be progressive, static, or remitting. The most common type of dementia is Alzheimer's disease, which affects approximately 2-4% of people older than age 65, and 20% of people over age 85. More than 4 million Americans currently are afflicted with Alzheimer's disease (Fendrick & Langa, 2002). Alzheimer's disease causes gradual death of brain tissue, which is believed to be related to chemical changes inside individual brain cells. Alzheimer's disease is not the only type of dementia; however, cerebrovascular accidents (strokes), arteriosclerosis (hardening of the arteries), alcoholism, vitamin deficiencies, serious head injuries, infections including human immunodeficiency virus (HIV), and other brain assaults (such as seen in an overdose or severe hypoxia) may also cause dementia. Neurological disorders, such as Parkinson's disease and Huntington's chorea, may progress to dementia symptoms in late stages. The recently publicized "Mad Cow Disease" (Creutzfeldt-Jakob disease) is a dementia related to a parasitic organism, as is end-stage syphilitic dementia. Pick's disease is characterized by a deterioration of the frontal lobe of the brain, with early personality changes as a prominent feature.

Other changes associated with dementia may include impairment of spatial orientation, poor judgment, and poor insight. Clients may be unaware of the extent of their memory loss or other cognitive abnormalities. Occasionally disinhibited behavior occurs resulting in inappropriate language, ignoring societal rules, over-familiarity with strangers, or even dangerous behaviors. Agitation is common as the disease progresses along with anxiety, mood, and sleep disturbances. Delusions are relatively common — often paranoid or persecutory in nature. Hallucinations, particularly visual, occur with some frequency as well. Individuals with dementia are highly susceptible to developing delirium with even small changes in medications or physical health status.

Computerized tomography (CT) scans and magnetic resonance imaging (MRI) may reveal cerebral atrophy, ischemic areas of the brain, focal lesions, or hydrocephalus (fluid in or around the brain). Most differential diagnosing is focused on ruling-out other diseases before a diagnosis of dementia is made.

The *DSM-IV-TR* categorizes dementia as multiple disorders, with varied etiologies, all of which share common symptomatology. Dementia is broken down into 10 separate disorders with an 11th, "not otherwise specified" category for those symptoms that don't fit easily into 1 of the 10.

Dementia of the Alzheimer's Type

Dementia of the Alzheimer's type is gradual and involves progressive cognitive decline, not due to another neurological disorder or substance. Brain atrophy may be detected by CT or MRI scans. Postmortem microscopic examination usually reveals neurofibrillary tangles, plaques, vascular degeneration, neuron loss, and other cellular changes. There is a familial tendency of the disorder thought to be associated with chromosome traits. *DSM-IV-TR* diagnostic criteria for dementia of the Alzheimer's type are as follows:

1. The development of multiple cognitive deficits manifested by both

    a. memory impairment; and

    b. one (or more) cognitive disturbances

        i. aphasia

        ii. apraxia

        iii. agnosia

        iv. disturbance in executive functioning

2. The cognitive deficits causing significant impairment in social or occupational functioning, and there is a significant decline from a previous level of functioning

3. Gradual onset and continuing cognitive decline.

4. The deficits in criterion 1 are not due to

    a. other central nervous system conditions

    b. systemic conditions (infections, vitamin deficiencies)

    c. substance-induced conditions

5. The deficits not occurring exclusively during a delirium

6. Disturbance not better accounted for by another primary psychiatric disorder (such as major depression or schizophrenia)

Vascular Dementia

Vascular dementia (formerly referred to as "Multi-infarct dementia) is less common than dementia of the Alzheimer's type. The onset is typically abrupt, followed by a fluctuating course of deterioration with sporadic cognitive impairments. To diagnose of vascular dementia, there must also be evidence of cerebral or peripheral vascular disease. Longstanding arterial hypertension, as evidenced by elevated blood pressure, an enlarged heart, abnormal heart sounds, or even cerebral emboli may be present. A single cerebrovascular accident (CVA) does not usually result in dementia, rather the disorder occurs following a series of greater and lesser CVAs with cognitive deficits more specific to the areas of the brain affected.

CT scans and MRIs typically indicate the extent of damage to the brain in the form of lesions in white and gray matter and focal atrophy.

Electroencephalogram (EEG) findings may also support focal lesions. Laboratory tests and electro-cardiograms (EKG) are useful in detecting other, concomitant diseases that may contribute to the dementia (e.g., liver impairment, renal failure). *DSM-IV-TR* criteria for vascular dementia are as follows:

1. Criterion 1 following the same as those for Alzheimer's dementia

2. Criterion 2 following the same as that of Alzheimer's dementia

3. Focal neurological signs and symptoms or laboratory evidence indicative of cerebrovascular disease being present, and related to the disturbance

4. Deficits not occurring exclusively in the course of a delirium

Dementia due to HIV

Dementia due to HIV occurs as a direct result of HIV infection. Pathological findings post-mortem usually reveal multifocal destruction of the white matter of the brain and subcortical structures. There may be an elevation in proteins and white blood cells (WBC) in spinal fluid. Dementia due to HIV often presents with forgetfulness, slowness, poor concentration, and decreased problem-solving abilities. The client may present with apathy and social withdrawal. Delusions, hallucinations, or delirium may be present. Physical exams can indicate tremors, imbalance, ataxia (unsteady gait), hyperreflexia, and other "soft" neurological deficits. Children with HIV infection may also develop dementia, characterized by developmental delays, microcephaly (small brain), flaccidity, and calcifications in the basal ganglia.

Dementia due to Head Trauma

Dementia may occur as a consequence of a serious head injury. The cognitive impairments seen are directly related to the areas of the brain sustaining the damage. Post-traumatic amnesia is frequently present and is associated with memory impairment. Behavioral symptoms may include aphasia, problems with attention span, anxiety, irritability, depression, or mood swings. Changes in personality are often seen. Dementia due to head trauma is not usually progressive, but repeated injuries (such as those seen in the sport of boxing), may lead to further deterioration (pugilistic dementia). This disorder is most often seen in young men who engage in risk-taking behaviors. Substance abuse or dependence should also be evaluated.

Parkinson's Disease

Parkinson's disease is a slowly progressing neurological condition associated with lowered dopamine levels in the brain. It is characterized by tremors, rigidity, bradykinesia, and unsteadiness. Dementia occurs in Parkinson's disease at a rate of 20-60% — usually in more advanced cases. Gradually diminishing executive functioning, forgetfulness, and impaired memory occur in conjunction with the motor symptoms of this disease. Parkinson's disease may occur in addition to Alzheimer's disease or vascular or other dementias.

Huntington's Disease

Huntington's disease (also referred to as Huntington's chorea) is an inherited disorder transmitted equally in men and women, and a result of a single autosomal dominant gene on the short arm of chromosome 4. Symptoms usually begin between age 30-40; however, both juvenile-onset and late-onset cases have been noted. Early symptoms are elusive and include personality and behavior changes, depression, anxiety, and irritability. Motor symptoms present as fidgeting, then progress to a full lack of motor control. Cognitive changes of impaired memory, decreased judgment, and altered executive functioning occur early in the disorder, with progressive deterioration including disorganized speech and even psychosis (hallucinations and delusions). Children of individuals with

Huntington's disease have a 50% chance of inheriting the disorder.

Pick's Disease

Pick's disease is a degenerative disease of the brain that specifically affects the frontal and temporal lobes. Personality changes occur early in the course of the illness, with behavioral disinhibition, deteriorated social skills, language abnormalities, and emotional blunting occurring. Other criterion-1 features of dementia occur later. Primitive reflexes (e.g., sucking, grasping) may occur. Apathy or extreme agitation may occur as the disease progresses. Brain imaging may reveal frontal or temporal lobe atrophy. Pick's disease commonly occurs in clients between age 50-60.

Creutzfeldt-Jakob Disease

Dementia due to Creutzfeldt-Jakob disease is a disorder that is the direct result of the presence of spongiform encephalopathies, a group of central nervous system diseases caused by agents known as prions, or "slow viruses." These agents are transmitted via infected brain tissue. Cases have been documented related to bovine (cattle) transmission through tainted meat, and recently deer have tested positive for the prions. There have also been reports of transmission secondary to corneal transplantation and human growth factor injections. Individuals with Creutzfeldt-Jakob disease usually experience fatigue, anxiety, problems with appetite or sleeping, or poor concentration early on, progressing to poor coordination, altered vision, and abnormal gait or other motor movements. The dementia onset is fairly rapid — usually over the course of a few months — and criterion-1 symptoms are present. Up to 25% of clients may have an atypical presentation, and the diagnosis can only be verified at autopsy. The transmissible agent is resistant to ultraviolet radiation, boiling, alcohol, or formalin, but it is susceptible to pressurized autoclaving and chlorine bleach.

Other Dementia Disorders

Other dementia disorders may occur as a result of numerous medical conditions. Table 5-1 presents an overview of some additional dementia disorders. To make the diagnoses, criterion 1 and 2 must be met, as well as a preponderance of evidence from the history, physical examination, or laboratory findings that the dementia is the direct result of the medical condition.

Substance-induced persisting dementia is a dementia disorder that requires that both criterion 1 and 2 are met, and that there must be evidence from the history, physical examination, or laboratory tests that the deficits seen are etiologically related to persisting use of a substance, or exposure to a toxin. Delirium may be present, but the dementia symptoms must persist even when the delirium has resolved. Blood or urine drug screens may be negative. The age of onset is after 20, and can only occur after prolonged substance exposure. Substance-induced persisting dementia may be related to the following abused substances: alcohol, inhalants, sedatives, hypnotics, or anxiolytics; related to the following medications: anticonvulsants,

TABLE 5-1: MEDICAL CONDITIONS THAT MAY LEAD TO DEMENTIA DISORDERS							
Structural Lesions	**Endocrine Abnormalities**	**Nutritional Deficiencies**	**Infectious States**	**Organ Diseases**	**Neurological Disorders**	**CNS Injury**	**Rare Disorders**
Primary Brain Tumors	Hypothyroidism	Thiamine Deficiency	Neurosyphilis	Liver Failure	Multiple Sclerosis	Electrical Shock	Adult Storage Diseases
Secondary Brain Tumors	Hypoglycemia	Niacin Deficiency	Cryptococcus	Renal Failure	Status Epilepticus	Drowning	Childhood Storage Diseases
	Hypercalcemia	B$_{12}$ Deficiency	Prions			Intracranial Radiation	

methotrexate; or related to the following toxins: lead, mercury, carbon monoxide, organophosphate insecticides, industrial solvents.

Dementia disorder, not otherwise specified, is the term used for a dementia that does not meet criteria for any of the other disorders. It is commonly used when there is insufficient evidence to determine a more specific type.

THE MINI-MENTAL STATE EXAM

The Mini-Mental State Exam is a structured instrument originally developed in 1975 for the purpose of assessing an individual for the presence or absence of a dementia disorder. It is in widespread use today, many versions of which are developed in a convenient, pocket-sized tool. The Mini-Mental State Exam takes approximately 10-15 minutes to administer, and it can be administered by any health care provider. Several cognitive domains are assessed, including memory, language, orientation, apraxia, attention, and concentration. Items are scored one point for each correct answer with a total of 30 possible points. A score below 23 usually indicates dementia, although scores from 23-26 may suggest a well-compensated dementia disorder as well. Clients should be assessed in a quiet environment with the health care provider's full attention. Table 5-2 provides some sample items from the Mini-Mental State Exam.

COMMONLY PRESCRIBED MEDICATIONS FOR DEMENTIA

There is no known cure for dementia. The neurotransmitter acetylcholine (ACh) is involved with memory and cognitive abilities in the brain. Alzheimer's dementia appears to selectively dam-

---

TABLE 5-2: MINI-MENTAL STATE EXAM SAMPLE ITEMS

Orientation to Time
"What is the date?"

Registration
"Listen carefully, I am going to say three words. You say them back after I stop.

Ready? Here they are...

HOUSE (pause), CAR (pause), LAKE (pause). Now repeat those words back to me."

[Repeat up to 5 times, but score only the first trial]

Naming
"What is this?" [Point to a pencil or pen]

Reading
"Please read this and do what it says." [Show examinee the words on the stimulus form.] CLOSE YOUR EYES

---

age neurons that produce and distribute ACh (Agronin, 2002).

The 1970 cholinergic hypothesis of Alzheimer's disease postulated that an ACh deficiency in the brain causes the cognitive impairments to be seen. One solution, then, was to inhibit the enzyme acetylcholinesterase (AChE) that breaks down ACh, leading to elevated ACh levels in the brain. AChE medications will not cure dementia or reverse the symptoms from already damaged neurons, but they do have usefulness in slowing the progress of the disease. AChE medications have also been linked to improved functioning overall and lowering behavioral problems. AChE medications include the following:

1. Reminyl® (falantamine) — inhibits AChE as well as binding to both presynaptic and postsynaptic nicotinic receptor sites that promote the

release of AChE. Prescribed up to 12 mg twice a day (b.i.d.).

2. Aricept® (donepezil) — perhaps the most frequently prescribed of the AChE inhibitors; side effects are low and easy to manage. Prescribed once a day up to 15 mg — usually at bedtime (h.s.).

3. Cognex® (tacrine) — rarely prescribed now due to an association with liver transaminase elevation in nearly 40% of patients. Prescribed up to a maximum of 40 mg four times a day (q.i.d.).

4. Exelon® (rivastigmine) — good AChE inhibitor similar to donepezil, but requires b.i.d. dosing. Prescribed up to a dose of 6 mg b.i.d.

Side effects of the AChE inhibitors may include gastric upset including nausea and/or vomiting, decreased appetite, weight loss, and diarrhea. Fatigue or insomnia may develop, and headaches are occasionally reported. Starting with a low dosage and titrating slowly will help to ameliorate many of these problems.

The AChE inhibitors are only indicated for Alzheimer's type dementia disorders. Other types of dementia may benefit but clinical studies have not yet supported this. Vascular and other medical-related dementias should be treated as appropriate for that disorder.

NURSING CARE OF THE CLIENT WITH DEMENTIA

Nursing care of the client with a dementia disorder reflects the areas of deficits observed. Assisting in the assessment process including administering the Mini-Mental State Exam, getting a good nutritional and substance abuse history, obtaining laboratory tests, and preparing clients for CT and MRI scans, and EEGs will facilitate a rapid and accurate diagnosis. Education is very important early in the disease process — both with the client and the family. A good working knowledge of community resources for caregivers of individuals with dementia disorders will provide invaluable information to the families. Many Internet resources are also available. Maintaining a sense of security and safety for the client becomes increasingly important as the disease state progresses. In late stages of dementia, a client will need assistance with basic care, such as bathing, dressing, and feeding. Mortality from dementia is secondary to other medical conditions including opportunistic infections. Keeping the client clean and comfortable, and providing support for families will help to ease their grief during terminal care.

In talking with a client with moderate to severe dementia, it is important to remember that the client may become easily frustrated and agitated. The client may make statements that are accusatory or hurtful in nature. It is important for nurses and family members alike to maintain a calm presentation and not allow personal anger or hurt feelings to affect judgment. Dementia is a progressive disorder. Teaching new information may be an unrealistic goal; in fact the client may be unable to remember information presented only a few minutes before including names. Repetition and patience are of utmost importance. It is fruitless to engage in a debate to "convince" a client with dementia of certain facts, rather the nurse should focus on underlying feelings and continuously reassure the client of his safety. Maintaining eye contact, moving slowly, and approaching the client from the front while repeating his name will help to diminish fear or startle the client. Choices and options should be upbeat, positive, and limited in range or demands. The nurse should speak slowly and clearly, using simple and easy to understand words. If a client is having difficulty in verbal expression (aphasia or dysphasia), it is useful to revert to close-ended questions that can be answered simply with a "yes" or "no" response — gestures, visual cues, and prompts will help as well. Changing the subject is a useful tool when a client is becoming clearly frustrated.

DIFFERENTIATING DELIRIUM FROM DEMENTIA

The essential feature of a delirium is a change in cognition that cannot be better explained by a preexisting dementia disorder, accompanied by an alteration in level and state of consciousness (*DSM-IV-TR*, 2002). There must be evidence from the history, physical examination, or laboratory tests that the symptoms exhibited are a result of a medical condition, substance use (or withdrawal), toxin exposure, or a combination of these factors. In delirium, there is a reduced awareness of others and the environment. Focus and attention are impaired, memory and perceptual experiences may be impaired, and disorientation (especially to time) is present. Language disturbances may be evident as well. The client may present as incoherent and/or agitated. Hallucinations are not uncommon along with illusions (misinterpreting items or people in the vicinity), and misperceptions (misunderstanding sights, sounds).

Delirium is often associated with alterations in the sleep-wake cycle. Increased motor activity in the form of restlessness, groping, picking at bedclothes, and sudden movements may occur. Sluggishness, lethargy, and near-stupor may also be seen. Emotional lability can range from fear to irrational anger to inappropriate giggling. Mood shifts can be rapid and unpredictable. Paranoia can lead to aggression or self-injury (falling out of bed, pulling out IV lines). Screaming, crying, calling out, cursing, moaning, and other vocalizations may be heard. Signs of autonomic hyperactivity (elevated heart rate, elevated blood pressure, diaphoresis, flushed face, and dilated pupils) are often present. In hepatic encephalopathy (related to liver disease) and other encephalopathies, a flapping movement of the hands known as "asterixis" may occur.

EEG readings are often abnormal, showing either fast activity or a generalized slowing. The symptoms of a delirium can develop over a few hours to a few days. Recovery is closely related to the underlying etiology.

The *DSM-IV-TR* differentiates five types of delirium: Delirium due to a general medical condition; delirium due to substance intoxication; delirium due to substance withdrawal; delirium due to multiple etiologies; and delirium, not otherwise specified.

Delirium due to a general medical condition must have demonstrated evidence of the medical condition, and the delirium must be etiologically related to that disorder. Diagnostic criteria include the following:

1. Disturbance of consciousness with a reduced ability to focus, sustain, or shift attention

2. Change in cognition (such as memory deficit, disorientation, language disturbance) or developing perceptual disturbance, which is not better accounted for by dementia

3. Disturbance developing over a short period of time (hours to days) and tending to fluctuate during the course of the day

4. Evidence from the history, physical examination, or laboratory findings showing disturbance resulting from the direct physiological consequences of a general medical condition

To diagnose a substance-induced delirium there must be evidence of substance intoxication, toxin exposure, or medication side effects (including drug interactions), in addition to criteria 1 through 3 noted previously. Substance-induced delirium often arises within minutes to hours of exposure to rapid-acting agents such as cocaine or hallucinogens. Onset can be delayed for longer-acting agents, which may only become toxic once elevated serum levels are reached (e.g., benzodi-azepines, such as diazepam, or poisons). Usually the delirium resolves once the offending agent is metabolized and excreted by the body (or dialyzed if necessary). Poor renal or hepatic function will slow resolution of the delirium. Certain medications commonly used in psychiatric care have narrow therapeutic ranges versus toxic dosing ranges, and clients may become delirious when overmedicated. These medications include lithium carbonate or lithium citrate, all of the tricyclic antidepressants (e.g., imipramine, desipramine, amitriptyline, nortriptyline) and valproic acid (Depakote®). Delirium is also frequently seen in the postoperative patient secondary to a combination of anesthesia effects and pain medications, or in individuals abusing high levels of opiate-based pain medications, benzodiazepines, or illicit drugs.

Withdrawal associated delirium occurs as when substances are cleared by the body. It's usually associated with longer half-life agents, or with agents that cause habituation through inducing liver enzymes (e.g., alcohol, diazepam, opiates). The onset and duration of the delirium is associated with the half-life of the agent. Alcohol withdrawal delirium may begin within 24 hours of the last drink, whereas diazepam (Valium®) withdrawal delirium may not start for 3-5 days.

Delirium due to multiple etiologies is seen when a client presents with a delirium, and there are numerous causative factors. An example of this would be a client with hepatic encephalopathy who is also dependent on alcohol. *DSM-IV-TR* criteria 1 through 3 remain the same, criterion 4 requires that there is evidence that the delirium has more than one etiology.

The term "delirium, not otherwise specified" (delirium, NOS) is used when there isn't yet enough evidence to support the diagnosis of an associated medical condition, substance intoxication, or substance withdrawal. It also includes delir-iums associated with unusual causes such as sensory deprivation.

THE TREATMENT OF AGITATED AND AGGRESSIVE CLIENTS

Care must be taken when treating a client who is agitated or aggressive. This behavior is commonly seen with delirium, and is often associated with dementia when the client is undergoing a stressor such as anxiety, fear, fatigue, insomnia, or a medical illness. The phenomenon of "sundowning" may occur with dementia as well. This involves an increasing confusion and agitation that starts in the late afternoon and becomes more severe as the night progresses. Dangerous behaviors such as wandering into the streets may occur. Nursing care should be focused on maintaining safety and providing reassurance and support. Medications need to be used cautiously so as not to increase the agitation or induce a worsened delirium.

Medications that have potent anticholinergic properties may increase disorientation and confusion. These include antipsychotics, tricyclic antidepressants, and antihistamines. Benzodiazepines (in low doses) are usually preferable for the acute treatment of a delirious patient. Medications such as buspirone (Buspar®) and trazodone (Desyrel®) are also useful. Administering an agent similar to the detoxifying substance, in smaller titrated doses can help in substance withdrawal delirium. Agitation associated with hallucinogen use can be managed with antipsychotics (while monitoring for emergent extrapyramidal syndrome side effects). New-generation antipsychotics are preferable as the risk for extrapyramidal syndrome is much lower than that of traditional antipsychotics.

One of the newer generation antipsychotics, ziprasidone (Geodon®), is now available in an intramuscular formulation. Besides having sedative properties, it also has efficacy for acute antipsychotic (reducing hallucinations and delusions) treatment.

Occasionally, physical restraints become necessary in the disoriented and agitated client. The health care provider should be trained in the proper application of the restraints so as to avoid harm to the client. Soft wrist restraints and vest restraints are preferable to leather restraints. The client should be monitored frequently while in restraints, and there needs to be documented evidence of nursing checks for skin injuries or bruising, opportunities for fluid and nutrition, and opportunities for bowel or bladder elimination. Restraints should be removed as soon as the agitation is reduced to a level that is determined to no longer present a risk to the safety of the client or others.

DEMENTIA CASE STUDY

Chip is a 72-year-old man who is living with his adult daughter and her family. His family physician suspected dementia when Chip began having difficulty in finding his way home from the grocery store. A neurology consult and MRI scan provided further evidence to support the disorder, and the neurologist prescribed Aricept® 10 mg a day. Most of the time, Chip is oriented to his surroundings and pleasant and cooperative with his family. He has been having increasing problems in the evening with confusion and recently became quite agitated and left the house at 11:00 p.m. "to go to work". Chip is a retired telephone lineman. After one of these episodes, his family physician prescribed 100 mg of amitriptyline (Elavil®) at bedtime in an attempt to help him sleep better. Three nights after taking this medication, Chip became extremely agitated and was yelling out, "Get them out of here! Get those men away from those lines before they blow!" His family had to call an ambulance to get him transported to the emergency department where he was sedated and then admit-

ted to the medical-psychiatric unit. His admitting diagnoses were substance-induced delirium, and dementia of the Alzheimer's type. Elavil® was discontinued and in 2 days he was able to return home to his family.

NURSING CARE PLAN

Problem Listing

• Potential for injury

• Fear

• Family support needed

Nursing Diagnoses

1. Risk for injury related to drug toxicity as evidenced by acute delirium and agitation.

2. Fear secondary to a belief in threat or harm as evidenced by delusional statements.

3. Caregiver role strain related to increasing illness of client as evidenced by progressive dementia and attempts to leave the house.

Long-term Goal

Both client and family will receive the level of support needed to ensure ongoing positive relationships while maintaining a high standard of safety.

Short-term Objectives

1. Client will not sustain injury during period of delirium.

2. Client will demonstrate reduced fear by displaying a calmer demeanor and following simple directions.

3. Family will report an increased level of satisfaction with community resource awareness and availability by the time client is ready for discharge.

Nursing Interventions

1. Staff will monitor client closely and administer medications p.r.n.

2. Staff will assess for the need of temporary, soft wrist restraints during the acute phase of the agitation and delirium.

3. Staff will administer fluids and maintain a patent IV line.

4. Staff will use a soft, comforting voice tone and inform client of his safety during all procedures.

5. Staff will allow family members to remain at bedside as desired during hospitalization period.

6. Staff will provide social service resources and information on local caregiver support programs to family prior to client's anticipated discharge date.

EXAM QUESTIONS

CHAPTER 5
Questions 30-36

30. A required criterion to diagnose a dementia disorder is

    a. the presence of neurofibrillary tangles in the brain.

    b. a fluctuating course of disorientation.

    c. decreased problem-solving abilities.

    d. an impairment in memory.

31. Dementia of the Alzheimer's type has a

    a. rapid onset and rapid decline in functioning.

    b. gradual onset and continued decline in functioning.

    c. gradual onset with no decline in functioning.

    d. rapid onset with no decline in functioning.

32. Essential factors that differentiate a delirium from dementia include

    a. a disturbance in consciousness with a gradual onset and a declining course.

    b. extreme disorientation and delusions without a change in consciousness.

    c. a gradual onset of confusion and depressive symptoms.

    d. a disturbance in consciousness with a fairly rapid onset and a fluctuating course.

33. A medication group that may precipitate a delirium even at therapeutic or recommended doses in a susceptible client is

    a. antibiotics.

    b. tricyclic antidepressants.

    c. selective serotonin reuptake inhibitors.

    d. multivitamins.

34. *Charlie is a 52-year-old man who is arrested with a Breathalyzer test of .26 for public intoxication. He is incarcerated until his family can be found to bail him out. 48 hours after his arrest, he tells the jail matron that his skin is crawling and he keeps seeing spiders crawling across the ceiling. Within 4 hours, the staff find him screaming incoherently and cowering in the corner. He looks "twitchy," sweaty, and flushed.*

    The most likely cause of these symptoms is

    a. untreated paranoid schizophrenia.

    b. hallucinogen overdose (acquired from his cell mate).

    c. substance withdrawal delirium associated with alcohol dependence.

    d. a manipulative attempt to get out of jail and into a hospital.

35. A priority for nursing care of the client with either a dementia disorder or a delirium is

    a. promoting self-esteem.

    b. reorienting to reality.

    c. maintaining safety.

    d. educating about the illness.

36. The nurse working with a client who has a moderate degree of dementia should

    a. speak clearly and be prepared to repeat instructions patiently.

    b. educate the client thoroughly about his medications.

    c. expect clients to remember health care facility routines.

    d. encourage the family to institutionalize the client for safety.

CHAPTER 6

ALCOHOL AND SEDATIVE ABUSE AND DEPENDENCE

CHAPTER OBJECTIVE

At the end of this chapter, the reader will be able to discuss alcoholism and sedative, hypnotic, and anxiolytic dependence in American society including the recognition and treatment of withdrawal syndromes.

LEARNING OBJECTIVES

At the completion of this chapter, the reader will be able to

1. describe signs of alcohol and sedative, hypnotic, anxiolytic intoxication, and withdrawal.

2. discuss medical and nursing care for withdrawal from alcohol or sedative, hypnotic, and anxiolytics.

3. recognize medical disorders that are associated with alcohol dependence.

4. discuss therapy and family issues that occur in the alcohol-addicted client.

ALCOHOL DEPENDENCE

"We, of Alcoholics Anonymous, are more than one hundred men and women who have recovered from a seemingly hopeless state of mind and body...the only requirement for membership is an honest desire to stop drinking. We are not allied with any particular faith, sect or denomination, nor do we oppose anyone". This quote is from the first edition of the 1939 printing of *Alcoholics Anonymous: The Big Book* (1976). By 1955, membership in Alcoholics Anonymous (AA) had grown to over 150,000 individuals in nearly 6,000 groups, no longer located solely in the United States. By 1976, there were over 28,000 groups made up of over 1 million members.

Today, alcohol disorders are found in 7.4% of adults in the United States while drug abuse and dependence is present in 3.1% of adults. The health and societal costs attributed to alcohol-related illnesses, injuries, and deaths is astronomical with estimates at more than $100 billion annually. Alcohol dependence often has a familial pattern with a risk of developing a dependency 3-4 times higher in children of alcohol dependent persons over that of the general population. Contributing environmental factors may include cultural attitudes toward drinking, the availability (and legality) of alcohol, the effects of alcohol on mood and behavior, and perceived levels of stress (Keltner, Schwecke, & Bostrom, 2003).

ALCOHOL INTOXICATION

Alcohol intoxication is characterized by behavioral or psychological changes such as mood lability, mild euphoria, reduced inhibitions, impaired judgment, or aggression that develop shortly after ingestion of alcohol. Other symptoms may include slurred speech, poor coordination, unsteady gait, impaired memory, decreased attention span, nystagmus of the eyes, and even stupor or coma. The amount of alcohol required to produce these changes varies in an individual based on factors such as gender, age, body mass, and genetic vulnerabilities, but most healthy adults can metabolize approximately one drink (one beer, glass of wine, or "shot" of hard liquor) an hour. Impaired judgment begins at a blood alcohol level of 0.08-0.1%. "Blackouts," or episodes where the intoxicated individual is awake and functioning but has no memory of the time spent, usually occur at a high blood level in the occasional drinker, but may occur at a very low blood level in the alcohol dependent person.

Metabolism of alcohol occurs in the liver where it is broken down first into acetaldehyde and hydrogen, then into acetic acid, which later ends up as carbon dioxide and water. Acetaldehyde is toxic to the liver where it impairs normal cellular functioning, interferes with the absorption of vitamins, and increases fat storage. Tolerance to alcohol is probably associated with elevated liver enzyme levels and cellular adaptation.

ALCOHOL WITHDRAWAL

Alcohol withdrawal symptoms begin as soon as the body begins to metabolize the alcohol into acetaldehyde. Often these early symptoms are masked as the individual continues to imbibe. After a night of sleeping, a "hangover" may be experienced, which is characterized by irritability, headaches, nausea, vomiting, and dizziness. Repeated intoxication will lead to alcohol tolerance then dependence. Withdrawal effects for the dependent person will begin when the serum alcohol level begins to drop near zero, and the detoxification process may continue for 3-5 days. Table 6-1 presents an overview of initial, intermediate, and severe signs of alcohol withdrawal.

TABLE 6-1: ALCOHOL WITHDRAWAL SYMPTOMS (UNTREATED)

Initial
Elevated heart rate
Elevated blood pressure
Headaches
Mild nausea
Subjective sensations of anxiety or restlessness
Cravings
Sleep disturbances

Intermediate
Severe cravings
Hand or whole body tremors
Hot, flushed skin
Diaphoresis
Significantly elevated BP and pulse
Nausea, vomiting, diarrhea, stomach cramps
Dizziness or light-headedness
Dehydration (low grade temperature & thirst)
Irritability, hostility

Severe
Illusions or hallucinations
Delusions
Delirium
Panic level anxiety
Agitation or assaultiveness
Seizures (grand mal)
Any symptoms as noted above

Alcohol withdrawal management usually consists of liberal use of benzodiazepine agents as soon as symptoms are seen. An elevated blood pressure and pulse reading are the best indicators — although consideration should be made for the client with primary hypertension in which case an elevated pulse rate alone is a more sensitive measure. Benzodiazepines work to alleviate the associated anxiety and restlessness through a tranquilizing effect, and to reduce the risk of seizure development and delirium tremens, a psychotic state characterized by hallucinations (usually visual) and paranoid delusions. The more physiologically dependent a client is on alcohol, the more difficult and uncomfortable the detoxification period will be. Medications commonly used include lorazepam (Ativan®), chlordiazepoxide (Librium®), and diazepam (Valium®). Diazepam is particularly useful in the emergency department as it may be administered IV.

Cross-tolerance is a phenomenon where a client develops tolerance for agents similar to the drug-of-choice. It is not unusual to find a cross-tolerance effect between alcohol and benzodiazepines. The nurse may need to administer relatively high doses of benzodiazepines initially in the detoxification process to manage this problem. Other "comfort" medications may be given, such as promethazine (Phenergan®) for nausea and trazodone (Desyrel®) to aid in sleep. Acetaminophen should be avoided due to its extensive metabolism in the liver. Similarly, aspirin is contraindicated due to a risk of increased bleeding times associated with liver disease, as well as esophageal and gastric ulcerations. Ibuprofen is a better choice for minor aches and pains. Vitamin administration is usually an automatic part of alcohol detoxification — in particular the water soluble B-vitamins including thiamine, niacin, and folic acid — due to the metabolic problems with vitamin absorption in a fatty liver.

MEDICATIONS FOR ALCOHOL DEPENDENCE

No medications are indicated primarily to treat alcohol dependence; however, two agents may have some usefulness. Naltrexone (Revia®) is an opioid receptor site antagonist that reduces alcohol cravings. It is believed to block some of the pleasure responses induced by alcohol in the brain through occupying the endorphin receptors in the neurons. Naltrexone will induce immediate narcotic withdrawal in an individual who has been using opioids; therefore the health care provider needs to assess the client carefully for other substance

dependencies. Naltrexone has long been used in emergency care under the name Narcan® as a treatment for opioid (e.g., heroin, morphine) overdosage. Disulfiram (Antabuse®) is a drug that inhibits the breakdown of acetaldehyde in the brain. When alcohol is consumed in the presence of disulfiram, the individual experiences an immediate reaction, which may include symptoms such as flushing, sweating, nausea, vomiting, tachycardia, hypotension, headache, heart palpitations, tremors, and weakness. Disulfiram alone can be stressful on the liver, and monitoring of liver enzymes is recommended. Disulfiram and alcohol together can induce cardiac arrhythmias, seizures, myocardial infarction, and cardiac failure. The purpose of disulfiram is to act as a behavioral deterrent for the client. Presumably, when taking disulfiram, the client will be less likely to succumb to the desire to drink due to a fear of becoming ill.

A newer clinical approach has been to utilize selective serotonin reuptake inhibitors (SSRIs) in the treatment of alcohol-dependent clients. Drugs such as fluoxetine (Prozac®), sertraline (Zoloft®), paroxetine (Paxil®), and escitalopram (Lexapro®) have shown some usefulness in helping to alleviate both depressive and anxiety symptoms in alcohol-dependent clients. It is unclear as to whether the substance abuse is a contributing factor to the mood symptoms, or whether the mood problems are a result of the substances themselves; however, most clients report improved moods and decreased relapse-inducing cravings when they are taking SSRIs. Additionally, SSRIs are nonaddictive, easy to dose, and relatively low in side effects.

MEDICAL COMPLICATIONS OF ALCOHOL DEPENDENCE

Alcohol is a central nervous system (CNS) depressant. Every year young men and women die of alcohol poisoning, from ingesting amounts of alcohol that are too much for the liver to metabolize before respiratory suppression and cardiac problems result. Alcohol is also a vasodilator, which predisposes individuals to frostbite and death from hypothermia. The combination of alcohol and other substances can be particularly lethal.

Alcoholic hallucinosis is a condition that may be experienced by the alcohol dependent client. In alcoholic hallucinosis, the client develops psychotic symptoms (hallucinations and delusions) while intoxicated. Psychosis can also occur during alcohol withdrawal, commonly known as delirium tremens.

Wernicke-Korsakoff syndrome is an alcohol-induced, persistent dementia disorder characterized by memory deficits, a foggy or clouded consciousness, peripheral neuropathies, and often confabulation (making up events or answers to fill in memory gaps). Wernicke-Korsakoff syndrome is closely related to thiamine and niacin deficiencies in the brain, along with chronic toxicity secondary to acetaldehyde.

Administration of B-complex vitamins and thiamine injections at the time of detoxification may help to reverse some of the cognitive problems, but the dementia experienced is usually irreversible.

Liver disease (fatty liver, cirrhosis) leads to obstructed blood flow through the liver. This causes portal hypertension, ascites (fluid in the abdominal cavity), and esophageal varices (swelling of the arteries supplying blood to the esophagus). Ascites put pressure on the diaphragm and make breathing more difficult. Esophageal varices may rupture and cause death by exsanguination (bleeding) or asphyxiation. Decreased liver functioning contributes to prolonged blood clotting time, elevated ammonia levels in the serum, elevated bilirubin levels, and low albumin (protein) levels, and predisposes the individual to confusion, jaundice, malnutrition, and edema.

Alcohol is an irritant to tissues and mucous membranes. As an irritant, the stomach responds by increasing production of hydrochloric acid, which then results in gastric and duodenal ulcers. Hemorrhage from ulcers can be dangerous if not life threatening.

A variety of other medical complications may develop associated with alcohol dependence. Thiamine deficiencies also contribute to peripheral nervous system problems experienced as chronic pain and a "tingling" sensation in the extremities. Pancreatitis and diabetes mellitus are seen at higher rates in the alcohol dependent client. Skeletal and cardiac muscle damage may occur leading to myopathies and enlargement of the heart. Night vision and peripheral vision may be reduced by damage to the eyes. Prolonged alcohol abuse in men decreases testosterone levels and may result in impotence.

Alcohol use during pregnancy, especially in the first trimester, can result in fetal alcohol syndrome. Infants born with this disorder often have varying degrees of mental retardation. Physical defects may or may not be present. Two key characteristics of fetal alcohol syndrome seem to be poor social skills and a high level of impulsivity in behaviors. The ability to distinguish between right and wrong (moral development) is also often impaired.

THE AA MODEL

A physician named William Silkworth first conceived the idea of AA in 1935 following the treatment of a stockbroker from New York. The stockbroker described a spiritual epiphany as instrumental in his recovery. The stockbroker shared his recovery story during a business trip with a physician in Akron, Ohio, who was also an alcoholic. He stopped drinking as well, and the concept that one alcoholic could help another was born. The basic tenets of moral inventory, confession of personality defects, restitution to those harmed, helpfulness to others, and the belief in and dependence upon a higher power, still make up the AA model today. AA meetings are supportive in nature. There is not an identified leader (although members may choose to help organize meetings). Sharing is on a first-name only basis. Testifying, or telling one's story, is encouraged. Members are encouraged to deal with life "one day at a time," and tokens are given out for number of days of sobriety. Members further along in their recovery process are encouraged to become "sponsors" for new members. A sponsor's role is to be available for support and to give advice during times of vulnerability or temptation. The AA model is structured around 12 steps to recovery; in fact, various support groups are now often referred to as "12-step programs" in deference to the success of the AA model. These 12 steps are as follows:

1. To admit that we are powerless over alcohol and our life has become unmanageable

2. To believe that a Power greater than ourselves can restore us to sanity

3. To make a decision to turn our will and our lives over to the care of this higher Power

4. To make a searching and fearless moral inventory of ourselves

5. To admit to our higher Power, ourselves, and to another human being the exact nature of our wrongs

6. To be ready to have our higher Power remove all these defects of character

7. To humbly ask Him to remove our shortcomings

8. To make a list of all persons we harmed, and become willing to make amends to them all

9. To make direct amends wherever possible, except when to do so would injure the other person(s)

10. To continue to take personal inventory and admit when we are wrong

11. To seek through prayer and meditation to improve our conscious contact with our higher Power, and for knowledge and strength to carry out His will

12. To carry the message to other alcoholics, and to practice these principles in all of our affairs (*Alcoholics Anonymous: The Big Book,* 3rd ed., 1976)

STAGES OF CHANGE MODEL

In 1982, psychologists James O. Prochaska and Carlo DiClemente developed the Stages of Change Model (a.k.a., the Transtheoretical Model) to try and explain why individuals had so much difficulty in giving up cigarette smoking. Six distinct phases were identified. Today, these stages are recognized and taught in other forms of substance dependence including alcoholism (University of South Florida, 2003).

The Stages of Change Model is as follows:

Precontemplation

In this stage, individuals are not even thinking about changing their addictive behaviors. They may not believe it is a problem, or they may feel that others are unnecessarily concerned. Precontemplation is associated with four broad rationales: reluctance, rebellion, resignation, and rationalization. Reluctant individuals do not want to consider change; rebellious precontemplators do not like to be told how to act, and they want to make their own decisions; resigned persons feel overwhelmed by the problem and have given up hope; and rationalizing precontemplators have many reasons why the substance isn't really a problem in their lives.

Contemplation

In this stage, the individual is ready to consider the possibility that a change may be necessary. There is often a high level of ambivalence, and change is not yet assured. The health care provider can assist the person in weighing the pros and cons of making a change.

Preparation/Determination

The preparation stage signals the beginning of a commitment to change. Individuals begin to research options and gather information, such as calling treatment providers or reading Internet resources.

Action

Individuals in this stage are able to implement plans to make changes. Success is not guaranteed, but they have moved closer to their goals by making some definitive decisions and acting on those choices.

Maintenance (Relapse and Recycling)

During the maintenance stage, individuals may go through a series of relapses. Building new patterns of behavior is difficult and can be emotionally charged; change can take up to 6 months to complete. Family dynamics and relationships with friends are all affected. Relapsing in and of itself is a learning experience — individuals can be helped by learning "triggers" to relapse and how to substitute other activities in the future.

Termination

The final stage of change is referred to as termination. In this stage, the addicted person no longer finds that the substance is a temptation. Kern (2003) discusses transcendence as a consequence of termination. Transcendence refers to a final phase where the individual no longer uses the substance, and even feels that the "old life" has been left behind, replaced by a new way of living. The idea of relapse and substance abuse is foreign to this "new life" and would feel inappropriate or even bizarre.

TREATMENT INTERVENTIONS AND FAMILY ISSUES

Therapeutic Interventions

Treatment for alcoholism (and other drug dependencies) begins even before the acute detoxification period. An "intervention" may be the first step to recovery. In an intervention, selected family, friends, and significant others come together in a supportive setting (usually the client's home) and confront the client about the alcohol or drug usage, and how it has negatively impacted each of the people in the room. Interventions are highly emotionally-charged events and are best when facilitated by a trained specialist. After the people in the room express themselves, the target client is given an opportunity to respond. An intervention is not completed until a plan is in place for the next step, which is usually some type of detoxification program. At the end of the intervention, the client should feel supported by family, friends, and significant others and not abandoned or rejected.

Treatment Programs

Following detoxification, clients experience a wide range of emotions and treatment options. Intensive programs (24-hour facilities, 12-hour day programs) are geared to immersing in the recovery process by allowing the client to essentially suspend normal daily activities, such as employment or school, and to focus on education, self-awareness, and recovery. Intensive outpatient programs usually run 2-3 hours, three times a week and they may follow the residential or day programs. Intensive outpatient programs allow the client to gradually reintegrate into normal activities while still maintaining a pronounced emphasis on recovery. Weekly groups and individual therapy sessions may follow intensive outpatient programs. Cognitive behavior (or rational-emotive) therapists work to help clients to understand the events, behaviors, and thoughts that led to drinking (or drug-using) occurrences, then to "unlearn" these self-destructive patterns and replace them with more adaptive strategies. Cognitive behavior therapy is covered more thoroughly in Chapter 8: Major Depression and Related Disorders.

Family Issues

Children of alcoholics often grow up to become alcoholics or drug abusers, or to marry individual's with addictions. Many theories exist as to why this occurs — certainly, human beings are drawn to others with whom they feel familiar, but there may be deeper psychological drives in place (e.g., a need to repair childhood traumas through rehearsal and repetition). Family studies suggest pronounced genetic and familial inheritance factors with alcoholism as well. Breaking the pattern of addictions within a family requires a tremendous amount of awareness and patience. Children of addicted parents are more likely to be abused or neglected, or to end up in foster care or residential placements (due to their own behaviors, or to the incarceration or residential treatment of their parents). Clients who use alcohol or other substances to excess have little time left over for partnership or parenting responsibilities. Family life is almost always disrupted and chaotic. Numerous supports programs exist which include Children of Alcoholics (COA), Adult Children of Alcoholics (ACOA), Al-ANON, and Codependents Anonymous (CA), and families should be encouraged to attend the program appropriate for them. Codependency is a recognized phenomenon where the nonusing partner or spouse of an addict behaves in ways that subtly allow the addiction to continue, such as lying to the client's employer about not showing up to work, making excuses for negative behaviors to others (e.g., "Mommy's sick" when the addicted person has a hangover, or "You didn't mean to hit me, it was the alcohol talking!"), or even purchasing alcohol or drugs for the client with illogical rationales such as "He'll get it somewhere,

it might as well be at home." Codependent partners need to be helped to realize the part they play in encouraging the addictive behavior to continue. Family therapy may be essential in rebuilding trust and positive relationships within the family.

SEDATIVE, HYPNOTIC, AND ANXIOLYTIC ABUSE AND DEPENDENCE

Benzodiazepines, benzodiazepine-like substances, barbiturates, and barbiturate-like substances make up the class of sedatives, hypnotics, and anxiolytics. This class includes all prescription "sleeping pills" and all prescription antianxiety agents with a benzodiazepine-like action (buspirone is not included). Drugs with important other uses, such as antiepileptics, may also be included depending upon their abuse and dependence potential. Similar to alcohol, these categories of substances are CNS depressants. They may be prescription or "street" acquired. All can cause tolerance, dependency, and withdrawal syndromes. CNS depressants are extremely dangerous if taken in an overdose, especially if combined with other medications, street drugs, or alcohol. Table 6-2 presents an overview of sedative, hypnotic, and anxiolytic drugs commonly seen. One particular benzodiazepine — flunitrazepam (Rohypnol®) — has been labeled the "date rape" drug because of its potent sedative and amnesic actions. It is not legally available in the United States.

Benzodiazepines and barbiturates work by enhancing the effects of the neurotransmitter gamma-aminobutyric acid (GABA). The action of GABA is to open chloride channels at the cellular level, which make a neuron less responsive to other neurotransmitters such as serotonin, norepinephrine, and dopamine. The overall effect is a slowing down of neuron firing. Benzodiazepines and barbiturates contribute to this brain-inhibition effect and slow down excitability, agitation, nervousness, and

TABLE 6-2: SELECTED SEDATIVES, HYPNOTICS, AND ANXIOLYTICS

Classification	Generic Name	Trade Name	Common Usage	Comments
Benzodiazepines	alprazolam	Xanax®	Anxiolytic	Duration 2-4 hrs.
	oxazepam	Serax®	Anxiolytic	Duration 1-2 hrs.
	lorazepam	Ativan®	Anxiolytic	Duration 4-6 hrs.
	diazepam	Valium®	Anxiolytic, status epilepticus	Duration 10-12 hrs.
	clonazepam	Klonopin®	Anxiolytic, epilepsy, bipolar disorder	Duration 10-12 hrs.
	chlordiazepoxide	Librium®	Anxiolytic, alcohol detoxification	Very long half-life
	clorazepate	Tranxene®	Anxiolytic	Seldom used
	estazolam	Prosom®	Sedative, hypnotic	Newer on market
	temazepam	Restoril®	Sedative, hypnotic	Duration 8-12 hrs.
	flurazepam	Dalmane®	Sedative, hypnotic	Long duration
	triazolam	Halcion®	Sedative, hypnotic	Assoc. w/ psychosis
	flunitrazepam	Rohypno®	Sedative, hypnotic, amnesic	Illegal in U.S.
Non-benzodiazepine	zolpidem	Ambien®	Sedative, hypnotic	Less dependency
	zaleplon	Sonata®	Sedative, hypnotic	Less dependency
Chloral derivation	chloral hydrate	Noctec®	Sedative, hypnotic	Short-term use only
Barbiturate	secobarbital	Seconal®	Sedative, antiepileptics	
	pentobarbital	Nembutal®	Sedative, antiepileptics	Dental anesthetic
	amobarbital	Amytal®	Sedative, amnesic, anesthetic	"Truth serum"
	butabarbital	Butisol®	Sedative, antiepileptics	
	phenobarbital	Luminal®	Antiepileptic, sedative	
	thiopental	Pentothal®	Anesthetic, sedative	Used freq. in surgery
	methohexital	Brevital®	Anesthetic, sedative	
Miscellaneous	meprobamate	Equanil®, Miltown®	Anxiolytic, sedative	High abuse potential
	methaqualone	Quaalude®	Sedative, hypnotic	High abuse potential

(often) alertness, attention span, concentration, and decision-making abilities. GABA receptors are located on approximately 40% of all neurons. GABA receptors are required for benzodiazepines to have an inhibitory effect. Barbiturates both enhance and imitate GABA, so receptor availability is not as important. Of the two groups, barbiturates are far more lethal than benzodiazepines (Keltner et al., 2003).

The *DSM-IV-TR* identifies four key criteria for identifying intoxication secondary to a sedative, hypnotic, or anxiolytic.

1. Recent use of the sedative, hypnotic, or anxiolytic.

2. Significant maladaptive behavioral or psychological changes that develop during or after use.

3. One or more of the following signs:
   a. Slurred speech
   b. Incoordination
   c. Unsteady gait
   d. Nystagmus of the eyes
   e. Impaired memory or attention
   f. Stupor or coma

4. The symptoms are not due to a general medical condition or another mental disorder.

Intoxication signs and symptoms of a sedative, hypnotic, or anxiolytic are almost identical to those of alcohol and differentiation should be made using a Breathalyzer® or blood alcohol test. In the presence of a sedative, hypnotic, or anxiolytic, a urine drug screen will test positive for benzodiazepines or barbiturates.

SEDATIVE, HYPNOTIC, AND ANXIOLYTIC WITHDRAWAL

The timing and severity of withdrawal syndromes are positively correlated with the pharmacokinetics and pharmacodynamics of the substance used. Withdrawal from short-acting agents (e.g., alprazolam) can begin within hours. Withdrawal from longer agents (e.g., clonazepam) may not begin for 1-2 days, or even longer. Withdrawal symptoms may include the following:

increased heart rate; increased blood pressure; sweating; hand tremor; insomnia; nausea or vomiting; visual, tactile, or auditory hallucinations; agitation; anxiety, including panic attacks; and grand mal seizures. Withdrawal from benzodiazepines and barbiturates often requires medical intervention and supervision. Administering gradually decreasing doses of the offending agent, or a similar substitution is accepted practice. Detoxification may occur in either an inpatient or an outpatient setting; however, in an outpatient setting the client must exercise a great deal of self-control and discipline to maintain the weaning schedule. The more rapid the weaning schedule is, the more uncomfortable and potentially dangerous it may be for the client. A weaning schedule of up to 2 weeks (sometimes longer) is recommended.

NURSING CARE OF THE CLIENT DETOXIFYING FROM ALCOHOL, SEDATIVES, HYPNOTICS, OR ANXIOLYTICS

Recognition of the signs of withdrawal and appropriate treatment is foremost when caring for a client withdrawing from alcohol, sedatives, hypnotics, or anxiolytics. Often, protocols are in place that allow the nurse to medicate the client based on set criteria, such as blood pressure and pulse. Ignoring the client's objective symptoms, or subjective complaints will result in a worsening of withdrawal symptoms and a potential for seizure. In the first 1-2 days of detoxification, fairly liberal use of withdrawal agents is recommended. Seizure precautions are an important safety measure due to the risk of neuron excitability. Assessing the client for other medications that may lower seizure threshold is important (e.g., buproprion, traditional antipsychotics, clozapine). Other safety concerns include monitoring for the emergence of psychotic symptoms, agitation, aggression, or suicidal thoughts and treating as necessary. Clients who present already well into withdrawal complications may require physical restraints for protection of themselves and the health care providers. Supporting fluid and electrolyte status through both oral and intravenous routes may be necessary. Administering a bland diet and antiemetics will help in controlling nausea and vomiting. Encouraging the client to maintain bed rest as much as possible for the first 24 hours will aid in the recovery process. It may be necessary to limit visitors in an inpatient setting to facilitate a quiet and nonstressful environment. Assessing for, and assisting in the treatment of, concomitant medical problems should be ongoing.

Assessment Tools

Assessment tools are useful to guide the health care provider in determining the severity of the use, making an appropriate formal diagnosis, planning treatment, and in monitoring ongoing progress. Most assessment tools are simple, standardized questionnaires that can be self-administered or administered by a health care provider; more than 100 such tools are available, many of which are free of charge. The Clinical Institute Withdrawal Assessment Scale (CIWA) is an 8-item instrument that can be administered and scored in less than 10 minutes. The CIWA is useful for clinical quantification of the severity of the alcohol withdrawal. It is available from the Ventana Clinical Research Corporation in Toronto, Canada (phone 1-416-963-9338) at no cost, or at www.niaaa.nih.gov. Similarly, Paolo DePetrillo and Mark McDonough developed the Alcohol Withdrawal Syndrome Type Indicator in 1999 in order to provide a simple assessment tool for alcohol withdrawal syndrome (AWS) symptoms. The AWS Type Indicator uses a simple "yes" or "no" rating scale and it divides withdrawal symptoms into three subtypes: A, B, and C. Subtype A (4 items) addresses CNS excitation symptoms, such as anxiety, restlessness, or hypersensitivity to light and sound.

Subtype B (7 items) evaluates adrenergic nervous system activity including nausea or vomiting, tremors, sweating, blood pressure and heart rate readings, and apical pulse irregularities. Subtype C (9 items) assesses signs of delirium including confusion, disorientation to person-place-time, and psychosis. The AWS Type Indicator takes about 3 minutes to administer. It is available free of charge for noncommercial use from the Focused Treatment Systems at www.sagetalk.com (or by calling 1-800-728-6799).

Once the acute phase of detoxification is completed, client education becomes extremely important. Both clients and their families or significant others need to understand the dynamics of addictions and addictive behaviors. A nonjudgmental approach, with practical and supportive information is most useful. Discharge planning will include referrals to outpatient treatment providers as well as AA or NA (Narcotics Anonymous). Many outpatient programs exist ranging from once-weekly therapy, to group therapy three times a week (Intensive Outpatient Program), to residential care with 12 hours of programming daily.

ALCOHOL DEPENDENCE CASE STUDY

*M*aggie is a 38-year-old woman who has been employed as a real estate agent for the past 10 years. She graduated high school and completed 4 years of a business degree before landing this lucrative position for a large company. In high school, Maggie drank some with her friends. She had her first blackout at her senior prom — later she found out that she was dancing on the tables and making a fool of herself. In college, she attended various fraternity parties and had another blackout episode. This time she awoke to find herself naked and in bed with two men. She had no memory of the preceding events. Maggie continued to drink socially on weekends, and then she started

taking prospective customers out during the week. Soon she found herself having wine with lunch, a cocktail or two after work, then several more in the evening at home. After Maggie's mother suddenly died of an aneurysm, her drinking escalated further to the point that she started to call in sick to work or go home early. She got her first DUI arrest while driving back to the office after showing a house. Her second DUI arrest (while at work) 2 months later cost her both her job and her driver's license. Unemployed, her drinking started to spiral out of control and she was always either intoxicated or sick. One night, Maggie started to vomit blood in copious amounts. Frightened, she called 911 and was rushed to the emergency department where she had surgery to repair a ruptured esophageal varicocele. She was detoxified after 5 days, and started attending AA meetings while in the hospital. Maggie learned that she was an alcoholic, and would always be an alcoholic. She agreed to see a therapist and continue to attend AA meetings once discharged. Maggie relapsed three more times before she was able to reach 2 years of sobriety and become a sponsor for another woman.

NURSING CARE PLAN

Problem Listing

- GI bleeding
- Poor nutrition
- Ineffective coping
- Insomnia
- Alcohol withdrawal: tremors, dizziness, diaphoresis, elevated BP and heart rate
- Anxiety

Priority Nursing Diagnosis

Potential for harm due to alcohol withdrawal as evidenced by tremors, elevated vital signs, anxiety, diaphoresis, and dizziness.

Long-term Goal

Client will be safely detoxified in a medically supervised setting.

Short-term Objectives

1. Client will have a consistent BP reading of less than 130/90.

2. Client will have a heart rate reading of less than 100.

3. Client will report less anxiety and fewer tremors.

4. Client will not develop hallucinations or other signs of psychosis.

Nursing Interventions

1. Assess BP, heart rate, and respirations every 2 hours and p.r.n.

2. Administer ordered benzodiazepines liberally every 2 hours and p.r.n.

3. Administer antiemetics as needed.

4. Encourage sipping of electrolyte replenishing fluids continuously.

5. Monitor intake and output.

6. Assess for blood in emesis or in stools.

7. Provide a bland, light diet for the first 48-72 hours of detoxification (unless NPO).

8. Keep environment quiet and nonstressful by turning down lights, keeping temperature at a comfortable level, and keeping noise to a minimum.

9. Restrict visitors if necessary.

10. Provide emotional support to client and family.

11. Once first few days of detoxification are complete, educate client as to processes of alcohol addiction (tolerance, dependence, withdrawal).

12. Make referrals to appropriate agencies including AA meetings.

EXAM QUESTIONS

CHAPTER 6
Questions 37-42

37. Alcohol detoxification can last up to

    a. 6-12 hours.

    b. 1-2 days.

    c. 48-72 hours.

    d. 3-5 days.

38. The set of symptoms indicative of sedative intoxication is

    a. restlessness, pacing, rapid speech.

    b. perceptual alterations, euphoria.

    c. slurred speech, impaired memory, unsteady gait.

    d. a sense of peacefulness, relaxation, increased appetite.

39. A nursing safety concern paramount in both alcohol and sedative, hypnotic, and anxiolytic detoxification is

    a. preventing the development of seizures.

    b. educating families and clients.

    c. providing thorough discharge referrals.

    d. administering antiemetics and a bland diet.

40. Medications commonly used to treat withdrawal symptoms such as tremors, anxiety, and an increased seizure risk are

    a. benzodiazepines.

    b. antidepressants.

    c. anticholinergics.

    d. opiate receptor antagonists.

41. A medical complication caused by portal hypertension is

    a. esophageal varices.

    b. gastric ulcers.

    c. pancreatitis.

    d. peripheral neuropathies.

42. Family members of the alcohol addicted client

    a. are generally mentally healthy and well-adjusted.

    b. can develop alcohol or drug addictions as well.

    c. should separate from the alcoholic client as soon as possible.

    d. have no impact on the recovery process.

CHAPTER 7

SUBSTANCE ABUSE
AND DETOXIFICATION

CHAPTER OBJECTIVE

At the end of this chapter, the reader will be able to discuss drug dependency in American society including the recognition and treatment of withdrawal syndromes.

LEARNING OBJECTIVES

At the completion of this chapter, the reader will be able to

1. recognize signs of substance abuse and dependence.

2. differentiate symptoms of intoxication and withdrawal in opioids, amphetamines, cocaine, inhalants, hallucinogens, and nicotine.

3. discuss medical and nursing treatment for substance withdrawal.

SUBSTANCE ABUSE AND DEPENDENCE

The *DSM-IV-TR* differentiates substance abuse from substance dependence and substance-related disorders (which may include heavy metals, pesticides, poisons, or over-the-counter agents). The essential feature of substance abuse is a maladaptive pattern of substance use that is associated by recurrent and significant negative consequences related to the use of the substance. There must be repeated use during a 12-month period, which results in a failure to fulfill major role obligations at work, school, or home; or use in situations in which it is dangerous or hazardous (e.g., operating a motor vehicle); or substance-related legal problems such as arrests; or persistent social or interpersonal problems caused by the substance use. Substance dependence incorporates the criteria for substance abuse, but also requires that at least three of the following criteria are met.

1. Tolerance
   a. A need for increasing amounts of the substance to achieve intoxication; or,
   b. Markedly diminished effect with continued use of the same amount of the substance.

2. Withdrawal
   a. A withdrawal syndrome characteristic to the substance used; or,
   b. The substance, or a closely related substance, is taken to relieve or avoid withdrawal symptoms.

3. The substance is often taken in larger amounts or over a longer period than was intended.

4. There is a persistent desire or unsuccessful efforts to reduce or control substance use.

5. A great deal of time is spent in activities necessary to obtain the substance, use the substance, or recover from its effects.

6. Important social, work, or recreational activities are given up or reduced because of substance use.

7. The use is continued despite knowledge of having a physical or psychological problem that was likely caused or exacerbated by the substance.

Substance withdrawal syndromes are currently recognized for alcohol; amphetamines and related substances; cocaine; nicotine; opioids; and sedatives, hypnotics, and anxiolytics. Withdrawal develops when the amount of substance used is reduced or discontinued. Caffeine, nicotine, and marijuana have no clinically recognized withdrawal syndrome; however, symptoms are consistently reported and will be discussed in this chapter.

The use of multiple substances will complicate the clinical picture significantly and safe detoxification may be difficult.

OPIOID ABUSE AND DEPENDENCE

Opioids include commonly prescribed pain medications (both oral and intramuscular), intravenous drugs used on the streets, and certain anesthetics. Examples of opioid substances include opium, heroin, methadone (Dolophin®), morphine, codeine, hydromorphone (Dilaudid®), meperidine (Demerol®), hydrocodone (Lortab®), and oxycodone (OxyContin®, Percodan®, Percocet®, Tylox®). Opioids work by stimulating naturally occurring endorphin receptor sites in the brain and producing an overall sense of euphoria accompanied by an increased tolerance to pain and reduced anxiety. Side effects of opioids include drowsiness, respiratory depression, constipation, decreased gastric secretions, urinary retention, hypotension, and pinpoint pupils. An excess amount of opioids (overdosage) will produce central nervous system (CNS) depression, seizures, respiratory depression, stupor, coma, and possibly death. Naltrexone (Narcan® or Revia®), an opioid antagonist, is used to treat opioid overdose (Keltner, Schwecke, & Bostrom, 2003). Taking opioids with other CNS depressants, such as alcohol, benzodiazepines, or barbiturates, is especially lethal. Urine drug screens will test positive for opioid-like substances, which will assist in determining other drugs that may also be present.

Children born to women who are addicted to opioids will experience withdrawal symptoms at birth, which may include respiratory depression, irritability, tremor, diarrhea, and vomiting. Sudden infant death syndrome (SIDS) has been associated with heroin exposure prenatally. The neonate may initially suffer from Failure-to-thrive, but rarely are there any long-term medical or developmental complications. Information is not available on learning disabilities or other less overt problems that may emerge later.

Opioid Withdrawal

The *DSM-IV-TR* identifies the following criteria as necessary in determining opioid withdrawal:

1. At least one of the following:
   a. cessation or reduction of opioid use that has been heavy and prolonged; or,
   b. administration of an opioid antagonist after a period of opioid use

2. Three or more of the following, developing within minutes to several days after use is stopped, or after an opioid antagonist is administered:
   a. dysphoric mood
   b. nausea or vomiting
   c. muscle aches
   d. lacrimation (tears) or rhinorrhea (runny nose)
   e. pupillary dilation, piloerection ("goosebumps"), or sweating
   f. diarrhea
   g. yawning
   h. fever
   i. insomnia

3. The symptoms in criterion 2 causing significant distress or impairment

4. The symptoms not occurring due to a general medical condition or another mental disorder

Nursing Care of the Client with Opioid Withdrawal

Nursing care should be focused on supporting the client and providing reassurance. Opioid intoxication and overdosage is life threatening, but withdrawal is rarely dangerous unless other medical conditions are present. It is, however, uncomfortable for the client. Administering nonsteroidal analgesics such as ibuprofen will help with the muscle aching and leg cramps reported. Nonaddictive sleep aides such as trazodone (Desyrel®) are also useful. Monitoring and maintaining fluid and electrolyte status, as well as urinary output and bowel functioning, will help to avoid complications.

Monitoring visitors may be required with clients detoxifying from opioids. The desire to use ("cravings") can be overwhelming, and clients may make elaborate arrangements to obtain drugs to alleviate their symptoms. Some clinicians may prescribe clonidine (Catapres®, Catapres-TTS®) in oral or topical form. Clonidine is an alpha-adrenergic agonist that reduces impulses in the sympathetic nervous system resulting in a decrease in blood pressure, heart rate, and cardiac output, and prevention of pain signal transmission, anxiety, and hyperactivity. Another medication that may help to prevent relapse is buproprion (Wellbutrin®, Zyban®). Buproprion increases the amount of dopamine, serotonin, and norepinephrine in the brain, which appears to reduce cravings associated with substances such as opioids, cocaine, and nicotine.

COCAINE AND AMPHETAMINE USE

Cocaine is found naturally in the leaves of the coca plants. It was introduced to the West as an anesthetic in the mid-1800s. Cocaine was once used in soft drinks (Coca-cola®), but its use was eliminated in 1906. Cocaine is a powerful stimulant with significant euphoria, associated with its actions to block the reuptake of the neurotransmitter dopamine in the brain. Cocaine also depletes the neuronal stores of norepinephrine causing an adrenalin-like rush. Cocaine rapidly crosses the blood-brain barrier and is rapidly metabolized by the healthy liver resulting in a short length of action (2-4 hours). Effects of cocaine use include an increase in alertness, strength and endurance, sexual stimulation, motor activity, heart rate, and blood pressure. There is a decreased need for sleep and appetite is reduced. Inhibitions are also reduced. Because of its extensive abuse, medical uses of cocaine have ceased to be practiced. A relatively new form of less expensive cocaine is available on the streets. Mixing cocaine with baking soda and water, then heating it and allowing it to harden produces "crack" cocaine. It can then be smoked for an immediate high, which is followed by a significant crash. The depression experienced may lead to suicide attempts. "Crack" is considered one of the most addictive substances available (Keltner et al., 2003).

Amphetamines have been available since the late 1800s and have a variety of legitimate medical uses including the treatment of obesity, attention-deficit/hyperactivity disorder, and narcolepsy. Recently, amphetamines have been publicized more due to the accepted use of "Go Pills" in U.S. Air Force pilots with long flight assignments. All therapeutic amphetamines are administered orally, however illicit uses may include sniffing or intravenous use. Amphetamines include such substances as Dexedrine® (dextroamphetamine), Adderall® (mixed amphetamine salts), Desoxyn® (methamphetamine), and related substances Ritalin® (methylphenidate) and Ecstasy. Amphetamines may also be "cooked up," or produced in a homemade lab, making products such as "crank," "crystal meth," or "CAT" (methcathinone). Amphetamines are sometimes combined with heroin and injected in a "speed ball" — a particularly lethal combination. Amphetamines work by causing the release of norepinephrine and dopamine from nerve endings and blocking their reuptake, resulting in higher norepinephrine and dopamine brain levels. Side effects of amphetamines include alertness, improved concentration, increased energy, restlessness, insomnia, decreased appetite, and mood changes.

Too much amphetamine or cocaine at one time, or chronic usage, may result in severe agitation, tachycardia, cardiac arrhythmias, hypertension, increased respirations, and psychosis. Paranoid delusions and visual hallucinations may occur. Death is usually due to sudden cardiac arrest (seen primarily after intravenous use). Long-term use may result in malnutrition, gastrointestinal problems, chronic insomnia, and anxiety disorders. Sniffing or "snorting" the drugs can cause nasal septum perforations and chronic nosebleeds. Intravenous use may result in phlebitis, cellulitis, and infections that can ultimately lead to gangrene and tissue necrosis.

Cocaine and Amphetamine Withdrawal

One of the main concerns with cocaine and amphetamine withdrawal is a "crash" in mood symptoms, probably related to the exhaustion of norepinephrine and dopamine transmitters. Depression and suicide ideation can occur and may last for several weeks. Safety of the client is a primary nursing concern. Other withdrawal symptoms include irritability, fatigue, insomnia or hypersomnia, nightmares, increased appetite, and psychomotor retardation or agitation.

HALLUCINOGENIC AGENTS

Hallucinogens are agents that induce hallucinations. Natural hallucinogens include psylocybin (hallucinogenic mushrooms), mescaline or peyote (derived from cactus), and marijuana (from the *cannabis sativa* plant). Synthetic substances include lysergic acid diethylamide (LSD), phencyclidine (PCP) or "angel dust," and Ecstasy (3,4-methylenedioxymethamphetamine or MDMA). Hallucinogens result in a heightened awareness of reality, followed by distorted perceptions then visual, auditory, or tactile hallucinations. Colors, tastes, and musical sounds may seem more intense or vivid. Time may seem to be slowed down or speeded up. Emotional sensations range from euphoria and a sense of peacefulness and wonder, to fear, panic, confusion, and paranoid reactions.

Mescaline and psylocybin have traditionally been used in Native American religious practices. Hallucinogenic effects last up to 12 hours for mescaline and 8 hours for psylocybin. In addition to hallucinogenic effects, they dilate the pupils and increase heart rate, blood pressure, and body temperature. Occasionally psylocybin will cause a skin tingling sensation and involuntary movements.

Marijuana cultivation has taken place for over 5,000 years. It varies in potency dependent on soil and growth conditions, and varieties harvested. The active ingredient in marijuana, tetrahydrocannabinol (THC) is stored in fatty tissues in the body for up to 6 weeks after use. Marijuana is typically smoked, though it can be ingested as well. Effects from smoking last 2-4 hours while effects from ingestion may last up to 12 hours. Marijuana produces a sense of well-being and relaxation. It increases hunger and has antiemetic properties as well, which is why it may be useful for individuals undergoing chemotherapy for cancer or HIV-related diseases. Marijuana has also been indicated in reducing intraocular pressure associated with glaucoma. Side effects of use include impaired short-term memory and concentration, dry mouth, sore throat, increased heart rate, bloodshot eyes, and dilated pupils. Smoking marijuana can lead to bronchitis. There is some evidence to support reduced testosterone levels and sperm counts.

Emotional reactions other than a mild euphoria may include anxiety, panic, and paranoia.

LSD was initially developed as a potential treatment for schizophrenia. It has potent serotonin binding effects and can cause dramatic hallucinations that last up to 12 hours. Side effects of LSD ingestion include tachycardia, increased blood pressure, trembling, dilated pupils, sense of unreality, perceptual alterations, confusion, impaired judgment, and synesthesia. Synesthesia is the hallucinatory experience that causes an individual to feel as though he can "smell" colors or "taste" music. Severe emotional reactions may occur including panic and paranoia. LSD intoxication has been attributed to a number of suicides.

PCP has been used traditionally in veterinary medicine as a tranquilizer and anesthetic. PCP can be taken orally, intravenously, nasally, or smoked. Effects last up to 8 hours after use. PCP causes an initial euphoria with perceptual distortions. Side effects include increased blood pressure and heart rate, staggering, vomiting, increased salivation, bizarre behaviors, and muscular rigidity alternating with violent outbursts. The aggression and strength of PCP users is legendary in emergency department settings. Another anesthetic, Ketamine® ("Special K") has also been used for its dissociative effects. Ketamine® has been implicated in date rapes due to its amnesic properties.

Ecstasy (MDMA) has been around since the 1900s when it was synthesized primarily as an adjunct to psychotherapy. Its common use is in nightclubs and "Raves." At low doses, it increases affection and a sense of closeness to others. Higher doses result in an amphetamine-like response with euphoria, increased sexuality, and disinhibition. Mild hallucinogenic effects may also occur. Side effects are amphetamine-like with teeth grinding, tachycardia, dry mouth, and decreased appetite. Memory impairment may also occur. Deaths have

been reported secondary to hyperthermia, dehydration, rhabdomyolysis, and renal failure.

Nursing Care of the Client Using Hallucinogens

Overdoses of hallucinogens are not usually fatal. Deaths occur secondary to dangerous or risk-taking behaviors. Suicides and homicides are most likely to be associated with LSD and PCP respectively. Nursing care should focus on maintaining a calm, quiet environment. Antipsychotics may be indicated for persistent hallucinations. Chemical and physical restraints may be necessary. Benzodiazepines are useful for reducing panic and anxiety.

Withdrawal Management

Hallucinogens do not produce any physiological dependence, although a hallucinogen persisting perception disorder ("flashbacks") may occur. This is defined by the *DSM-IV-TR* as a recurrence of disturbances in perception similar to those experienced while under the influence of the drug. The symptoms must cause clinically significant distress, and cannot be due to a general medical condition or other mental disorder such as schizophrenia. Episodes may occur repeatedly and they usually abate after several months.

Marijuana users may experience extreme irritability, insomnia, restlessness, and increased activity during withdrawal.

INHALANT ABUSE AND DEPENDENCE

Inhalants such as gasoline, glue, paint thinners, and hydrocarbons found in cleaning solutions, correction fluid, and spray-can propellants (as well as a variety of other substances) are inexpensive and readily accessible. This leads to their abuse in children as young as elementary school. CNS effects include dizziness, euphoria, slurred speech, lethargy, depressed reflexes, psychomotor retardation, tremor, muscle weakness, blurred or double vision, nystagmus, incoordination, stupor, and coma. Other effects may include respiratory problems, coughing, sinus discharge, mouth ulcers, nosebleeds, headaches, gastrointestinal problems, confusion, and a loss of appetite. Inhalants can cause both central and peripheral nervous system damage. Memory problems, decreased problem-solving abilities, generalized weakness, and peripheral neuropathies are prominent. Recurrent use may lead to hepatitis, cirrhosis, or renal failure. Sudden death can occur from respiratory or cardiovascular depression, acute arrhythmias, hypoxia, asphyxiation, or electrolyte abnormalities. The odor of paint or solvents may be detected on the individuals clothing or breath, or a rash may be present around the nose and mouth. There are no withdrawal symptoms (*DSM-IV-TR*).

CAFFEINE INTOXICATION AND WITHDRAWAL

Caffeine is an insidious and ubiquitous drug. It is legal and widely available in coffee, tea, chocolate, soft drinks, and new "energy "drinks. Caffeine is added to many over-the-counter drug products including some aspirins (Excedrin®), cold remedies and diet aids. Even caffeine tablets (No-Doz®) are easy to obtain. Table 7-1 provides an overview of some sources of caffeine along with average milligram dosages. All ages, even young children or infants consume caffeine.

Caffeine intoxication is characterized by at least five (or more) of the following symptoms that develop following the consumption of caffeine (*DSM-IV-TR*):

- restlessness
- nervousness
- excitement
- insomnia
- flushed face

TABLE 7-1: SOURCES OF CAFFEINE

Source	Dosage in milligrams
Coffee, brewed	100-140 mg per cup
Coffee, instant	65-100 mg per cup
Tea, black	40-100 mg per cup
Tea, green	30-50 mg per cup
Soda/soft drink	45 mg per 12 oz. can
Energy drinks	200-250 mg per can
Chocolate bar	5 mg per bar
OTC Analgesics	25-50 mg per tablet
OTC Cold remedies	25-50 mg per tablet
Diet Aids	75-200 mg per tablet

- diuresis
- gastrointestinal disturbance
- muscle twitching
- rambling flow of thought and speech
- psychomotor agitation
- tachycardia or cardiac arrhythmia
- periods of inexhaustibility

Most Americans consume approximately 200 mg of caffeine daily. Intoxication symptoms of rambling thoughts, psychomotor agitation, tachycardia, or arrhythmias usually occur at 1,000 mg or above, although symptoms may not be present if tolerance through repeated use has developed. Higher doses have produced ringing in the ears, flashing lights, severe headaches, and anxiety. Doses of 10,000 mg or more have resulted in grand mal seizures and respiratory failure leading to death (usually seen in overdoses).

A specific withdrawal syndrome is not identified by the *DSM-IV-TR*, however clients who abruptly stop caffeine use report problems with headaches, irritability, hypersomnia, fatigue, and hunger for 1-2 days after discontinuation.

Caffeine-induced sleep disorder typically produces insomnia at a dose-dependent effect (e.g., the higher the dose of caffeine, the worse the sleep problems). A client may experience insomnia secondary to caffeine even when other symptoms of caffeine use (alertness, increased energy) are not present.

NICOTINE DEPENDENCE AND WITHDRAWAL

Increased interest has been shown in the past few years to the issue of nicotine use and dependence. Nicotine dependence can develop with all forms of tobacco, and with prescription nicotine-withdrawal preparations (skin patch, gum). Nicotine dependence is associated with cardiovascular risk. Smoked nicotine (in the form of tobacco) is associated with diminished pulmonary function tests, cough, chronic obstructive pulmonary disease (COPD), lung and oral cancers, ulcers, and excessive skin wrinkling. The *DSM-IV-TR* recognizes nicotine dependence and withdrawal as a major health problem. Criteria for nicotine withdrawal include the following:

1. Daily use of nicotine for at least several weeks.

2. Abrupt cessation or reduction, followed (within 24-hours) by at least four of the following symptoms:
   a. dysphoria or depressed mood
   b. insomnia
   c. irritability, frustration, or anger
   d. anxiety
   e. difficulty concentrating
   f. restlessness
   g. decreased heart rate
   h. increased appetite or weight gain

3. The symptoms causing significant distress or impairment

4. The symptoms not occurring due to a medical or other mental disorder

Management of Nicotine Withdrawal

Withdrawal from nicotine, though uncomfortable, does not necessitate hospitalization. The reader is encouraged to review the 6 stages of change that an individual may experience discussed in Chapter 6 — a brief discussion of these stages follows. Precontemplation (stage 1) occurs when the client is not yet ready to change or wants to change. During contemplation (stage 2), individuals are thinking about their smoking, but have not yet made a commitment to stop. The preparation and determination stage (stage 3) begins the process of research into support and treatment programs for the client. Once ready, a plan of action is put into place (stage 4). Clients should be educated as to the detrimental effects of nicotine use, and then counseled on an ongoing basis to support efforts to stop. Use of nicotine transdermal skin patches, nicotine inhalers, and nicotine gums may assist in helping the client to overcome the smoking (or chewing) habit first, then gradually stepping down the dose of nicotine delivered later. Another alternative is to set up a "smoking schedule" where the client agrees to limit to smoking one cigarette an hour for several days, then one every 2 hours and so forth until discontinuing smoking entirely. Cognitive behavioral therapy is very beneficial; it helps the individual to recognize certain events or situations that trigger a desire to smoke, then to change those behaviors into actions that are less harmful. Maintenance of recovery (stage 5) can be extremely difficult and cigarette smokers may relapse repeatedly. Finally, termination (or transcendence) occurs when the client no longer desires or even wants to be around cigarette smoking or any form of nicotine use (stage 6).

SUBSTANCE DEPENDENCE CASE STUDY

Simon is a 40-year-old man with a long history of back problems. He was employed as a brick-

layer/hodcarrier for 20 years, and injured his back through repeated heavy lifting on the job. The resultant back spasms caused him to be bedridden for days to weeks at a time. In an effort to obtain relief, Simon's family physician placed him on muscle relaxants (Flexeril®) four times a day and gave him hydrocodone 5mg/acetaminophen 500 mg (Lortab® 5/500) tablets to take as needed. Simon had some initial pain relief, but soon found that the Lortab® "stopped working." He increased his dose to every 4 hours, and then he started to take 2 tablets at a time. He quickly ran out and his physician refused to prescribe more, but offered him a referral to a pain management clinic. Feeling somewhat desperate, Simon called his dentist to report chronic pain secondary to an infected tooth. The dentist called in a prescription for Percocet® until Simon could be seen. After getting the prescription, Simon cancelled the dental appointment. By now he was taking up to 30 tablets of painkiller a day — some were his wife's "old" prescriptions and some were purchased from friends. Simon also scheduled and kept appointments with four different physicians to have his back pain evaluation. All of them gave him pain pills — some with 2 or 3 refills. When Simon was near to running out, he would go to the local emergency department (ED) and invariably would receive a Demerol® injection and a prescription. This pattern of behavior continued despite family concerns until Simon began vomiting and turned sallow in color. He was again taken to the ED, but this time his diagnosis was acute hepatitis secondary to acetaminophen overdosage. In the ED, Simon was given Narcan® and had an nasogastric-tube placed for a stomach lavage. He was then hospitalized and placed on Mucomyst® every 4 hours around the clock for 3 days with BID acetaminophen levels and daily liver enzymes. Simon reported feeling "like I've been hit by a Mack truck." He was tremulous and diaphoretic. He alternated between chills and flushing. He experienced nausea, vomiting, diar-

rhea, muscle cramps, and back spasms so intense that he was in tears much of the first 2 days. After he became more medically stable, the physician prescribed Neurontin® for the chronic pain and gave him some ibuprofen for generalized discomfort and trazodone (Desyrel®) to aid in sleep. On discharge, a referral was made (and kept) to a pain clinic where Simon received physical therapy combined with steroid injections, topical analgesics (Lidocaine® patches), heat, massage, and education regarding the importance of activity and weight loss.

NURSING CARE PLAN

Problem Listing

- Chronic pain
- Inadequate coping responses to deal with pain
- Drug-seeking behaviors
- Opioid withdrawal symptoms
- Potential for injury
- Insomnia

Priority Nursing Diagnosis

Ineffective coping with chronic pain as evidenced by drug-seeking behaviors and opioid addiction.

Long-term Goal

Client will have minimal to no back pain without the use of addictive substances.

Short-term Objectives

1. Client will attend physical therapy appointments and practice exercises at home.

2. Client will verbalize an understanding of the dangers of overuse of prescribed medications.

3. Client will report a decrease in pain to a level that does not interfere with the enjoyment of life and daily activities.

Nursing Interventions

1. Educate the client and family as to the processes of addiction (tolerance, dependency, withdrawal).

2. Discuss with the client alternative pain management techniques that may be useful including heat, massage, gentle exercise, and stretching.

3. Facilitate education into alternate medication options.

4. Help the client to identify learned behaviors in response to pain.

5. Explain to the client that 100% remission is not the goal and help the client to identify what level of pain may be tolerable.

6. Assist the client in scoring or rating pain on a scale of 1-10 so that the client can better communicate how it feels to health care providers (and self).

7. Assist the client in identifying and listing diversional activities to use at home.

8. Teach the client relaxation techniques (breathing techniques) to be utilized when pain level is increasing.

43. One indication of substance dependence (as opposed to abuse) is that the client

    a. becomes intoxicated every weekend.

    b. demonstrates a need for increasing amounts of the substance to achieve intoxication.

    c. maintains a full-time job while using marijuana every evening.

    d. uses an amphetamine to stay awake and study for an exam.

44. Hallucinogens cause the following CNS responses

    a. dilated pupils, perceptual distortions, sense of unreality.

    b. euphoria, increased energy, hyperactivity.

    c. sluggishness, slowed hand-eye coordination, ataxia.

    d. improved concentration, increased alertness, insomnia.

45. An excess of amphetamines may cause

    a. stupor and coma.

    b. paranoid delusions and hallucinations.

    c. orthostatic hypotension.

    d. bradycardia and respiratory depression.

46. A characteristic of nicotine withdrawal is

    a. sluggishness and respiratory depression.

    b. decreased appetite, nausea, and vomiting.

    c. muscle aches, lacrimation, tremors.

    d. irritability, frustration, or anger.

47. A nursing safety concern during cocaine or amphetamine withdrawal is

    a. patient education.

    b. excessive sleepiness.

    c. malnutrition.

    d. suicide risk due to rebound depression.

48. *Tommy, a 10-year-old boy, comes to the health care facility for complaints of headaches, dizziness, and nosebleeds. He is noted to be staring off into space and he frequently answers questions with, "Huh?" or "What?" Tommy's mother is afraid he may have a brain tumor due to recent problems with forgetfulness and poor grades at school. There is a family history of alcoholism, and the parents are recently divorced. While checking his blood pressure, you notice a faint chemical odor.* Your nursing assessment should consider that Tommy

    a. may have a brain tumor and an MRI is needed stat.

    b. may have diabetes and the odor is from ketoacidosis.

    c. may be abusing inhalants and further evaluation is necessary.

    d. has poor hygiene and his mother is being overly dramatic and attention seeking.

49. In managing nicotine withdrawal, stage 4 involves

    a. precontemplating change.

    b. contemplating change.

    c. implementing a plan of action.

    d. maintaining remission.

CHAPTER 8

MAJOR DEPRESSION AND RELATED DISORDERS

CHAPTER OBJECTIVE

At the end of this chapter the reader will be able to identify symptoms of a depressive disorder and discuss relevant treatment including therapy and medications.

LEARNING OBJECTIVES

At the end of this chapter, the reader will be able to

1. describe the symptoms of depression.

2. differentiate major depression from other types of depressive disorders.

3. discuss various therapy modalities utilized when treating depression.

4. describe antidepressant medications and their side effects.

DEPRESSION

Depression is second only to hypertension as the most common chronic condition encountered in health care settings. Many cases are unrecognized or inappropriately treated, which may lead to lost wages, reduced productivity, declines in functional abilities, and poor physical health care and management (Whooley & Simon, 2000). Mortality associated with depression is significant with up to 15% of individuals suffering from recurrent depression committing suicide (Glick, 2002).

Suicide risk is highest in men who are over age 65, particularly if they are single, divorced, separated, or widowed. Suicide tends to be higher in Whites, with severe physical illness or substance abuse a contributing factor. Panic attacks and severe anxiety symptoms are also associated with increased suicides. Despite its relatively high prevalence rate (up to 10% in the U.S. population), depression continues to be stigmatized in our culture unless a person is perceived as having a "good reason" to be depressed (such as the loss of a job or death of a family member). Current psychiatric theories on the causes of depression certainly take into consideration environmental stressors, but neurobiological changes in the brain (particularly involving the transmitters serotonin and norepinephrine) have a significant impact on the severity and treatment responses of the disorder.

Five commonly recognized forms of depression will be discussed in this chapter: major depression, dysthymic disorder, seasonal affective disorder, premenstrual dysphoric disorder, and postpartum depression.

MAJOR DEPRESSION DISORDER

Major depression is characterized by a period of at least 2 weeks during which there is either a loss of interest or pleasure in nearly all activities, or there is a significantly depressed or irritable mood. Children and adolescents tend to experience grouchiness and irritability much more frequently than overt sadness. *DSM-IV-TR* criteria for major depression are as follows:

1. Five or more of the following symptoms have been present during a 2-week period and represent a change from baseline; at least one of the symptoms being (a) depressed mood (irritable in children and adolescents) or (b) loss of interest or pleasure:

   a. depressed or sad mood, may appear tearful (irritable mood in children and adolescents)

   b. loss of interest or pleasure in nearly all activities

   c. weight loss (without dieting) or weight gain (more than 5%), or a significant change in appetite

   d. insomnia or hypersomnia nearly every day

   e. restlessness/agitation or slowing/retardation observable by others

   f. fatigue or loss of energy

   g. feelings of worthlessness or excessive guilt

   h. difficulty concentrating or thinking clearly, or indecisiveness

   i. recurrent thoughts of death, suicidal ideation, or a suicide attempt

The symptoms must cause clinically significant distress for the client and interfere with their functioning in social or family, academic, or occupational areas. Major depression cannot be diagnosed during an expected course of bereavement unless the symptoms persist for longer than 2 months or are accompanied by marked impairments, morbid preoccupations, suicidal thoughts, psychosis, or severe psychomotor retardation.

The moods associated with major depression are often described as hopeless or feeling as if "in a black hole"; occasionally individuals report feeling numb or without emotion. Children may say that they never really feel happy, or that they think the family would be better off if they had never been born. Clients appear to stop caring about hobbies or social interactions, including with loved ones. Mild to moderate depression may stimulate the appetite in some clients and cause weight gain. Severe depression almost always results in a loss of appetite or complaints that food "tastes funny" or is without taste. Typical sleep disturbances with depression consist of normal to slightly delayed onset of sleep followed by middle of the night wakening. Sleep is described as "not restful" and children may report nightmares or be found wandering about the house. Fatigue and poor energy is pronounced. Thought changes include ruminations, obsessions, poor concentration, impaired decision-making abilities, worry, guilt, and occasionally psychosis. A phenomenon known as "pseudodementia" may occur during the course of a depression, particularly in older clients. Pseudodementia is the rapid onset of memory and concentration problems accompanying depression that may cause others to think that the client is developing a dementia disorder.

Psychotic symptoms occur in major depression up to 15% of the time (Glick, 2002). Clients who have psychotic symptoms during an episode of depression have a poorer prognosis than those who do not, and they may be indicative of the development of a bipolar disorder (especially when the symptoms are present in young children). Clients with a psychotic depression must be treated aggressively with antidepressants and antipsychotics due to the increased risk for harm to self or others.

Certain medications and medical conditions may aggravate or even trigger an episode of depression. Endocrine diseases such as hypothyroidism or diabetes mellitus can have a dramatic effect on moods and precipitate major depression, as can any disorder of the brain (dementia, epilepsy, multiple sclerosis, cerebrovascular accident (CVA), tumor), infectious or inflammatory dis-

TABLE 8-1: COMMON DEFENSE MECHANISMS

Defense Mechanism	Definition	Example
Repression	Involuntarily forgetting painful events.	A woman who was sexually abused as a child cannot remember it occurring.
Suppression	Voluntarily refusing to remember events.	An emergency room nurse refuses to think about the child who is dying of injuries from an auto accident.
Denial	Refusing to admit certain things to one's self.	An alcoholic man refuses to believe that he has a problem in spite of evidence otherwise.
Rationalization	Trying to prove one's feelings are justifiable.	A student insists that poor academic advising is the reason he cannot graduate on time.
Intellectualization	Using logic without feelings.	A father analyzes why his son is depressed without expressing any emotions of concern.
Identification	Attempting to model the self after an admired other.	Inner-city kids try to look and dress like a popular rap singer to feel stronger and more in control.
Displacement	Discharging pent-up feelings (usually anger) on another.	A child who is yelled at by her parents goes outside and kicks the dog.
Projection	Blaming someone else for one's thoughts or feelings.	A jealous man states his wife is at fault for his hitting her.
Dissociation	Unconsciously separating painful feelings and thoughts from awareness.	A rape victim "goes numb" and feels like she is outside of her body floating.
Regression	Returning to an earlier developmental level.	A 7-year-old child starts talking like a baby after the birth of a sibling.
Compensation	Covering up for a weakness by overemphasizing another trait.	A skinny, nonathletic kid becomes a chess champion.
Reaction formation	Acting exactly opposite to an unconscious desire or drive.	A man acts homophobic when he secretly believes he is gay.
Introjection	Taking on values, qualities, and traits of others.	A 12-year-old girl acts like her teacher when the teacher is out of the room.
Sublimation	Channeling unacceptable drives into acceptable outlets.	An angry woman joins a martial arts club and takes lessons.
Conversion	Converting psychiatric conflict into physical symptoms.	A lonely, elderly woman develops vague aches and pains all over.
Undoing	Trying to counteract or make up for something.	A man who yells at his boss sends her flowers the next day to "make up".

eases, electrolyte disturbances, severe nutritional deficiencies, toxins (such as lead or other heavy metals), alcoholism, and drug abuse. Many medications list depression as a possible side effect;

well-known problem medications include corticosteroids (e.g., prednisone), birth control pills, opioid pain pills, and some antihypertensives. An acne medication, Accutane®, has been implicated repeatedly in suicides of adolescents; however, clinical data has not yet been sufficient to have the U.S. Food and Drug Administration (FDA) remove it from the market. Antimalarial agents can precipitate both depression and psychosis in susceptible individuals, with reports of suicide attempts and violence. The Centers for Disease Control and Prevention recommends other antimalarial agents such as doxycycline for persons traveling to high-risk areas.

PSYCHOTHERAPY

Several psychotherapeutic models have been used in the treatment of depression. Until the advent of antidepressant medications in the 1950s, therapy was the sole treatment option. Clients could be depressed for periods of months to years. Today, therapy plus medication is the optimum management strategy resulting in episode durations of around 4-6 weeks in most cases (from the time of diagnosis).

Sigmund Freud the "grandfather" of psychotherapy, believed that depression and other psychiatric disturbances arose out of childhood experiences, and that the way human beings respond to their environment is based on unconscious drives or motivations. Freudian therapy (developed in 1936 and referred to as psychoanalysis) attempts to bring the unconscious into consciousness in order to allow individuals to work through past issues and develop insight into present behaviors. Perhaps the most practical application of Freud's teaching is the idea of defense mechanisms — or behaviors that an individual adopts in order to deal with stressors. Defense mechanisms can be beneficial and protective for the client, or counterproductive and

maladaptive. Table 8-1 provides an overview of commonly accepted defense mechanisms.

Another psychotherapeutic model used in the treatment of depression was developed in 1953 by Harry Stack Sullivan. He introduced the interpersonal model of therapy that considered psychiatric disturbances to be a disruption in the relationship between the individual and others. Therapy consisted of correcting the relationship defects to relieving anxiety and tension resulting in more mature, adult relationships. In order to do this, Sullivan incorporated the therapist as a tool by using sessions to present reality and validate or confront the client's beliefs. The therapist might make statements such as, "You say you're not angry, but I see you clenching your fists and hear you raising your voice." Interpersonal communication skills are taught to nursing students today, based on the early beliefs of Sullivan; a sampling of therapeutic and nontherapeutic communication techniques is provided in Table 8-2.

Cognitive behavior therapy has gained in both popularity and implementation in the past few years. Aaron Beck (1967) and Albert Ellis (1973) focused on the relationship between a client's perceptions about events and the resultant feelings and behaviors. This cycle of thoughts triggering feelings and behaviors is demonstrated in the following example:

Imagine you are driving down the interstate at 65 miles per hour. You look into your rear view mirror and see the flashing lights of a state trooper. Knowing that you are a little over the speed limit, you are certain he is pulling you over to give you a ticket. You think of the two glasses of wine you just had with dinner ("What if my blood alcohol level is too high? I can't be arrested! I would lose my job! They'll take away my nursing license!) You feel your palms get sweaty and your heart start to race. Barely able to contain your panic, you swerve quickly into the right-hand lane without signaling and cut off a car coming up behind you. The car honks, you get onto the shoulder and finally stop. In dread, you look out the window for the trooper. He continues past you down the highway.

In this example, the thoughts (*"I'm breaking the law by speeding,"* and *"I might get arrested for drunk driving."*) cause the driver to feel anxious and panic, which results in erratic behavior and nearly causes an accident. Now consider this example:

Imagine yourself driving down the interstate at 65 miles per hour. You look into your mirror and see the flashing lights of a state trooper. You know you're a little over the speed limit, but so is everyone around you. You think of the two glasses of wine you had with dinner, but you did eat a large portion and you don't feel drowsy — besides that was an hour ago. You deduce that there must be an accident fur-

ther down the road. You signal a right turn, check your mirrors and carefully pull over onto the shoul-der. After the trooper passes, you continue on your journey.

Cognitive behavior techniques are useful when treating a client with depression or an anxiety dis-order. Helping the client to identify beliefs (true or false) about situations will enable the client to chal-lenge those beliefs that are detrimental to recovery. Therapists who utilize cognitive behavior tech-niques are often quite structured with homework assignments each week. During each session, the therapist will review with the client specific situa-tions that occurred during the week and process the client's responses to those events. Role-playing may be employed. Some insurance companies have started to show preferential coverage for ther-

TABLE 8-2: THERAPEUTIC AND NONTHERAPEUTIC COMMUNICATION TECHNIQUES

Therapeutic Communication Techniques	Example
Asking an open-ended question	"How are you feeling?"
Offering self	"I'll sit here with you for a while."
Giving general leads	"Go on…you were saying."
Remaining silent	—— (sitting quietly)
Actively listening	Leaning forward, making eye contact, being attentive.
Restating	"So what you're saying is…."
Clarifying	"I don't quite understand. Could you explain…"
Making observations	"I notice that you shake when you say that."
Reflecting feelings	"You seem sad."
Encouraging comparisons	"How did you handle this situation before?"
Interpreting	"It sounds like what you mean is…"

Nontherapeutic Communication Techniques	Example
Asking a close-ended question	"Did you do this?"
Challenging	"Why did you do this?"
Arguing	"No. That's not true."
Not listening	Turning body away, making poor eye contact.
Changing the subject	[client states he is sad] "Where do you work?"
Being superficial	"I'm sure things will turn out just fine!"
Being sarcastic	"Just what do you mean by that, huh?"
Using cliché's	"All's well that ends well."
Being flippant	"I wouldn't worry about it."
Showing disapproval	"That was a bad thing to do."
Ignoring the client	"Did anyone read the paper today?"
Making false promises	"I'll make the doctor listen to you!"

TABLE 8-3: COMMONLY PRESCRIBED ANTIDEPRESSANT MEDICATIONS

Category	Generic Name	Trade Name	Sedation	Weight Gain	Ortho B/P risk	CNS Activation	GI Upset	Dry Mouth, Constipation, Urinary hesitancy	Comments
Tricyclic Antidepressants	amitriptyline	Elavil®, Endep®	+++	+++	+++	+	+	+++	Useful for chronic pain and fibromyalgia May ↑ Q-Tc delay
	nortriptyline	Pamelor®, Aventyl®	++	++	++	+	+	+++	May ↑ cardiac conduction delay
	imipramine	Tofranil®	++	++	++	+	—	+++	Used in enuresis in children May ↑ cardiac conduction delay
	desipramine	Norpramin®	++	++	++	+	—	+++	May ↑ cardiac conduction delay
	maprotoline	Ludiomil®	++	++	++	+	—	+++	May ↑ cardiac conduction delay
	clomipramine	Anafranil®	++	++	++	+	—	+++	May ↑ cardiac conduction delay
	doxepin	Sinequan®	+++	++	+++	+	—	+++	Highly sedating, Q-Tc delays
	protriptyline	Vivactil®	++	++	++	+	—	+++	May ↑ cardiac conduction delay
	amoxapine	Asendin®	++	++	++	+	—	+++	May ↑ cardiac conduction delay
	trimipramine	Surmontil®	++	++	++	+	—	+++	May ↑ cardiac conduction delay
Monoamine Oxidase Inhibitors	phenelzine	Nardil®	+	++	+++	+++	—	+++	Potent drug-drug interactions Dangerous drug-food interactions Can cause hypertensive crisis
	tranylcypromine	Parnate®	+	++	+++	+++	—	+++	Same as Nardil
	isocarboxazid	Marplan®	+	++	+++	+++	—	+++	Same as Nardil
	moclobemide	Manerix®	+	++	++	+++	—	+++	Little interaction with tyramine
Selective Serotonin Reuptake Inhibitors (SSRIs)	fluoxetine	Prozac®, Sarafem® Prozac® weekly	—	+	—	+++	+	—	First SSRI to be developed Longer half-life, very safe
	paroxetine	Paxil®	++	+++	—	+	+	++	More potent SSRI than Prozac
	sertraline	Zoloft®	+	+	—	++	++	+	Less potent, good in children
	citalopram	Celexa®	++	++	—	+	+	—	Mildly sedating, good HS
	escitalopram	Lexapro®	—	—	—	+++	+	—	Newest, very potent/activating
Miscellaneous Antidepressants	buproprion	Wellbutrin SR® Zyban®	—	—	—	+++	—	—	Acts on dopamine, stimulating Also used for smoking cessation
	venlafaxine	Effexor®, EffexorXR®	—	+	+	+	+	+	Both SSRI & TCA-like effects
	nefazodone	Serzone®	++	+	++	—	+	+	Watch for liver problems
	trazodone	Desyrel®	+++	+	++	—	—	+	Extreme sedation, good HS
	mirtazapine	Remeron®	+++	+++	—	—	+	+	↑ sedation, comes in dissolvable

+++ High   ++ Moderate   + Low   — Negligible

apists who use cognitive behavior techniques, as there is a good amount of data now supporting its treatment efficacy in as few as 6-8 sessions.

MEDICATION INTERVENTIONS

Four broad categories of medications are utilized in the treatment of major depression: tricyclic antidepressants, monoamine oxidase inhibitors (MAOIs), selective serotonin reuptake inhibitors (SSRIs), and miscellaneous agents. A discussion of each of these categories follows. Table 8-3 provides an overview of the most commonly prescribed antidepressants in these groups along with significant side effects or cautions. Adjunctive agents are sometimes necessary as well, of these the antipsychotic medications and mood stabilizers are the most common.

Tricyclic Antidepressants

Tricyclic antidepressants (TCAs) were the first medications developed to treat depression.

Imipramine (Tofranil®) was synthesized shortly after the antipsychotic chlorpromazine (Thorazine®) and it is similar both in molecular structure and side effects. TCAs work by blocking the reuptake of the neurotransmitter monoamines norepinephrine and serotonin, thus prolonging their activity in the brain. TCAs have a number of side effects. Sedation can be pronounced in some clients. In low doses, TCAs are useful for their sedative actions but clients may report worsened daytime fatigue and lethargy. TCAs also stimulate appetite and can cause weight gain. Central nervous system (CNS) side effects include tremors, potentiation of other sedatives, and cognitive clouding. Confusion and disorientation may occur, particularly in older clients. Clients can also exhibit pseudoparkinsonism symptoms such as those seen with traditional antipsychotic medications. Anticholinergic effects consist of dry mouth and eyes, urinary hesitancy, blurred vision, and slowing of the gastrointestinal (GI) tract leading to constipation. Cardiac and peripheral vascular effects can be pronounced with TCAs. Vasodilation can lead to orthostatic hypotension exhibited by dizziness, reflex tachycardia, and fainting. Delayed cardiac electrical conduction can lead to cardiac arrhythmias including premature ventricular contractions and ventricular tachycardia. Several deaths in children taking TCAs have been reported due to these arrhythmias. TCAs have a narrow therapeutic versus toxic range; monitoring serum levels is indicated. Other medications that are extensively metabolized similarly to TCAs (cytochrome P450, 2D6, 1A2 and 3A4 pathways) may have an additive effect and elevate blood levels of TCAs into a toxic range. Some of these medications include Tagamet®, Prozac®, traditional antipsychotics, quinidine, or other cardiac antiarrhythmics, levadopa, and some blood pressure medications. Using TCAs with monoamine oxidase inhibitors (MAOIs) is particularly dangerous. TCAs should be used cautiously in clients who have a history of suicide attempts or who are currently suicidal as they are highly toxic in an overdose.

Monoamine Oxidase Inhibitors

MAOIs, have been available almost as long as TCAs. Originally a derivative of the tuberculosis drug isoniazid, MAOIs work by inhibiting the enzyme that breaks down monoamines (serotonin and norepinephrine) thus making them more available in the brain. MAOIs are rarely used today due to extensive drug-to-drug and drug-to-food interactions. When MAOIs are taken in the presence of the amino acid tyramine (a product of tyrosine which is a precursor to dopamine, norepinephrine, and epinephrine) the client may experience a hypertensive crisis with BP readings upwards of 210/120. CVAs from hemorrhaging and death can occur. Foods that are high in tyramine levels are listed in Table 8-4. Drug interactions can be quite pronounced and the client should avoid all medications that have a stimulant activity (including over-the-counter cold remedies), SSRIs, TCAs, and numerous antihypertensives. CNS depressants may be intensified in the presence of MAOIs. Less dangerous side effects of MAOIs are related to increased activation in the brain. Clients complain of jitteriness, hyperactivity, anxiety, agitation, restlessness, insomnia, and euphoria. A drop in blood pressure normally occurs with MAOIs, for some clients this can be significant. Other side effects include dry mouth, blurred vision, constipation, and urinary hesitancy.

Selective Serotonin Reuptake Inhibitors

Selective serotonin reuptake inhibitors (SSRIs) have been the medications of choice for treating depression since fluoxetine (Prozac®) was first introduced about 15 years ago. SSRIs are effective and generally well tolerated by clients. They work by blocking the reuptake of serotonin (and other neurotransmitters to a lesser degree) in the brain's neurons. Most of them only require once a day dosing, and serum levels are not necessary due to

TABLE 8-4: FOODS HIGH IN TYRAMINE

Aged Cheeses and Milk

 Cheddar, blue, brie, mozzarella

 Sour cream

 Yogurt

Aged or Pickled Meats

 Bologna

 Liver

 Pickled herring

 Sardines

 Salami (luncheon meats)

 Most dried fish

Alcoholic Beverages

 Beer, alcohol-free beer

 Sherry wine

 Chianti wine

Fruits and Vegetables

 Bananas

 Figs

 Avocados

 Fava beans

 Sauerkraut

Miscellaneous

 Soy sauce

 Aged sauces

 Yeast

 Chocolate

 Licorice

 Caffeinated beverages

their relative safety in an overdose. SSRIs are mildly activating for most clients. Side effects include stimulation, insomnia, jitteriness, and stomach upset. Headaches and dizziness may occur. Some clients have sexual performance issues or decreased libido. Stimulants can potentiate the activating effects of SSRIs (including caffeine). A few of the SSRIs have some mild antihistamine-like activity that causes them to be sedating rather than stimulating, and to increase appetite (Celexa®, Paxil®). SSRIs are generally weight neutral — although some clients report a mild weight loss with Prozac® and weight gain with Paxil® and Zoloft®. SSRIs can have numerous drug interactions — in general they will potentiate the activity of medications that are highly protein-bound (e.g., TCAs) or that are extensively metabolized by cytochrome P450 (benzodiazepines, antipsychotics, some antihypertensives). Two serotonin-related syndromes have been identified: serotonin syndrome and serotonin withdrawal. Serotonin syndrome occurs when there is too much serotonin in the brain, as may be seen with certain drug interactions (MAOIs, St. John's wort) or in an overdose situation. Symptoms include restlessness or agitation, muscle twitching or jerking, sweating, shivering, tremors, abdominal cramps, diarrhea, nausea, headaches, ataxia, and hypomania or confusion/agitation. Serotonin syndrome is not life threatening. Treatment consists of stopping the medications and supporting metabolism with IV fluids. Serotonin withdrawal can occur when brain levels of serotonin are allowed to drop precipitously. Symptoms are described as flulike with dizziness, aching joints and muscles, a feeling of detachment, fatigue, and dizziness. Serotonin withdrawal occurs more predominantly with high-potency medications (Paxil®) and less with longer half-life products (Prozac®). Symptoms can be avoided by weaning off the medication over several days. Children rarely exhibit these problems. Serotonin withdrawal is uncomfortable, but not dangerous.

Miscellaneous Agents

Miscellaneous antidepressant agents are medications that have varied activity on neurotransmitters. Buproprion (Wellbutrin SR®, Zyban®) is a selective dopamine reuptake inhibitor. It is low in side effects with stimulation/activation being the chief complaint of clients. Mild increases in heart rate may occur. The primary concern with buproprion is that it lowers seizure threshold and may precipitate seizures in susceptible individuals. Buproprion should not be given to a client with epilepsy, an eating disorder, or during alcohol detoxification. Two interesting other actions of buproprion are that it reduces cravings (it's been approved for use in smoking cessation in the form of Zyban®), and it tends to increase libido (whereas SSRIs have a tendency to cause sexual dysfunction). Buproprion may be beneficial in treating attention-deficit problems as well.

Venlafaxine (Effexor®, Effexor XR®) is an antidepressant that acts like an SSRI in lower doses, but inhibits the reuptake of norepinephrine at higher doses. It is effective for chronic depression with an anxiety component. Side effects are low and primarily include GI upset. There have been some problems with venlafaxine elevating blood pressure in some clients, thus caution should be used in clients with primary hypertension.

Nefazodone (Serzone®) and trazodone (Desyrel®) are serotonin reuptake inhibitors plus receptor blockers. They are both good for depression associated with anxiety and insomnia. Trazodone is extremely sedating at therapeutic doses, so its usefulness is often limited to an adjunct treatment for depression-related insomnia. Trazodone can also cause the unusual side effect of priapism, which is a painful and persistent penile erection. Surgical intervention has been needed in some men. Nefazodone is well tolerated but has a number of drug-to-drug interactions along with a new, black box warning of risks for hepatic failure. A small percentage of clients cannot metabolize nefazodone well, and they experience a serotonin-like syndrome at low doses, or even with the initial dose.

Mirtazapine (Remeron®, Remeron SolTab®) works by blocking the feedback mechanisms for regulating serotonin and norepinephrine, thereby increasing their levels. It also has potent antihistamine activity. It is effective for insomnia and weight loss related to depression. Side effects other than sedation are quite low. Remeron SolTab® is a rapidly dissolving formulation that disintegrates on the tongue in less than 30 seconds. It is extremely useful in the extended care facility setting.

Adjunctive Medication Treatment

Adjunctive medication treatment may be needed when an antidepressant alone is insufficient. Clinicians may prescribe two antidepressants from different categories, in order to target the brain chemistry in as many ways as possible. An antipsychotic such as Geodon® can be quite helpful for severely treatment-resistant clients. Mood stabilizers (covered in Chapter 9) may be added including lithium carbonate and valproic acid (Depakote®). CNS depressants such as benzodiazepines may provide short-term anxiety relief, but excess use will result in cognitive dulling and potentially worsened depression. Medications are commonly prescribed for insomnia and may include trazodone, Ambien®, or Restoril®.

ELECTROCONVULSIVE THERAPY

Electroconvulsive therapy (ECT) is still a valid treatment option for the persistently depressed client who has not responded to antidepressant medications, or for whom antidepressant medications are contraindicated due to other medical conditions. During ECT, an electrical shock is passed through the brain for 0.2-8.0 seconds, causing a brain seizure. This induced seizure causes a flooding of neurotransmitters in the brain, which causes a more normalized pattern of electrical activity to occur (not unlike the effects in the heart following a cardiac defibrillation). It is not known how this neurotransmitter flooding alleviates depression, but clinical efficacy has been repeatedly demonstrated since the procedure was first developed in the early 1940s. Clients are given sedatives and muscle paralyzing agents, and breathing is supported. ECT is performed similarly to an outpatient surgical procedure, with preoperative and postoperative care. Treatments usually last less than 4 hours and are given 2-3 times a week for up to 12 treatments on an outpatient basis. With the use of medications, clients are no longer at risk for broken bones or injuries. Side effects of ECT are transient confusion after the procedure and memory impairments. Cardiac arrhythmias may also occur, which are thought to be related to a greater oxygen consumption of the skeletal muscles during ECT, resulting in ischemia to the heart in some clients.

DYSTHYMIC DISORDER

A dysthymic disorder is characterized as a chronically depressed mood nearly every day for over 2 years. Children may be irritable rather than sad (and the duration requirement is only 1 year). While depressed, at least two of the following other symptoms are present: poor appetite or overeating, increased sleep or insomnia, low energy or fatigue, low self-esteem, poor concentration or difficulty in making decisions, and feelings of hopelessness. Clients with dysthymic disorder are often self-critical and may see themselves as uninteresting. Dysthymic disorder is differentiated from major depression in that the intensity is less severe, the client may still be able to function in social, occupational, or academic areas, and there are no suicidal thoughts or urges. Dysthymic disorder is not diagnosed if there is a history of mania, or if the symptoms are associated with a psychotic disorder, substance abuse, a general medical condition, or a side effect of a medication.

Treatment for dysthymic disorder consists primarily of counseling (cognitive behavior techniques in particular) and antidepressant medications. SSRIs and miscellaneous agents are preferable due to their lower occurrence of side effects.

SEASONAL AFFECTIVE DISORDER

A seasonal affective disorder (SAD) is a depression that occurs primarily through the winter months. It tends to be more like a dysthymic disor-

der in severity; however, it may reach the level of major depression especially if there is a history of depressive disorders in clients or their families. SAD appears to be related to the hormone melatonin, which is produced by the body in response to sunlight. When melatonin levels are low, depression can result. The disorder is more prominent in the northern countries, and it occurs more frequently in women.

Treatment for SAD may include antidepressant medications, but clients may also choose to utilize full-spectrum light exposure through the use of special light bulbs designed for this purpose.

PREMENSTRUAL DYSPHORIC DISORDER

The criteria for a premenstrual dysphoric disorder (PMDD) are marked depressive moods, anxiety, and irritability with a decreased interest in activities that regularly occurs during the week prior to the onset of menses, and which are relieved when menses begins. The symptoms must be significant enough to interfere with functioning (work, school, other activities) and must be completely remitted for at least a week after the menstrual cycle. PMDD seems to be associated with sex hormones, in particular the rising progesterone phase of the menstrual cycle.

Initial treatment for PMDD may be the utilization of birth control pills or hormone replacement therapy to try and balance the estrogen and progesterone levels. If hormones are ineffective, poorly tolerated, or the client does not want to take them, then SSRI antidepressants are quite helpful. Fluoxetine in particular has been shown to be effective in treating PMDD and it is marketed under the name Sarafem® specifically for this purpose.

POSTPARTUM DEPRESSION

Depression with a postpartum onset occurs in the client within 4 weeks of the birth of the child. Postpartum "blues" are common and occur in up to 50-80% of new mothers (Keltner, Schwecke, & Bostrom, 2003). Postpartum depression is significantly more serious and may have an impact on the safety of the mother and infant. Infanticide can occur as a result of postpartum depression with psychosis; afterward mothers have reported that they believed their child to be possessed by demons, or that the child was doomed from the beginning. Postpartum depression with psychosis occurs in every 1 in 500-1,000 deliveries. Women with a history of major depression or previous postpartum depression are at the highest risk (30-50%) (*DSM-IV-TR*). Other behaviors toward the infant seen during episodes of postpartum depression may include disinterest, fearfulness of being left alone with the baby, anxiety, panic attacks, or overly-intrusive behaviors (such as waking the baby frequently). Prolonged depression in a new mother may be associated with problems in bonding with the child.

Treatment for postpartum depression starts with prenatal education. Expectant mothers and their families need to know that this is a real medical condition, and they need to be informed as to the symptoms that may be experienced (see criteria for major depression). If depression occurs, the mothers should be encouraged to seek treatment immediately, which may consist of a combination of therapy and antidepressant medications. Antipsychotics should be utilized for any psychotic symptoms. If the mother refuses to take medications, serious consideration should be made as to the safety of leaving the child in the home.

Clients with a history of major depression or postpartum depression should probably initiate antidepressant treatment during the third trimester of pregnancy. A study of 86 children (Nulman, Rovet, Stewart, Wolpin, Pace-Asciak, Shuhaiber, & Koren, 2002), looked at child development following prenatal exposure to both TCAs and fluoxetine and found that there were no significant deficits in cognition, language development, or the temperament of the children with mothers who took these medications. In fact, untreated depression in mothers was associated with less cognitive and language achievement in the children. Recommendations were that antidepressants be provided when needed during pregnancy.

NURSING MANAGEMENT OF DEPRESSIVE DISORDERS

Symptoms of depression affect nearly every body system, social relationship, and even an individual's personal sense or spirituality. Nursing care must be planned to take into consideration the whole client. Physical care may include treatment interventions to help alleviate insomnia or a loss of appetite. Diet education and nutritional supplements may be recommended. Clients who are depressed may not care for other medical conditions; therefore a thorough evaluation of these is necessary. Activities of daily living (ADLS) as basic as bathing and brushing one's teeth may be ignored by the severely depressed client. It is important to assist in structuring the client's day to try and maintain some contact with others, and some degree of cognitive stimulation. Safety should be assessed as suicide risk and other self-harm behaviors can be extremely high. It may be necessary to initiate an emergency detention and hospitalize a client who refuses treatment and is expressing suicidal ideation; hopelessness may cause the client to feel that there is nothing that can be done to help. Supporting and educating families is equally important. Depression can be very stressful on a family, and suicide is devastating.

Significant others should be educated that depression is a medical disorder and that there is effective treatment available. Family counseling may be necessary. Clients with depression who are employed may have medical leave benefits as well, which will help ease some of the financial pressures experienced by the family. Spiritual support, in the form of encouraging usual religious practices, can be helpful. Every effort should be made to allow hospitalized clients access to clergy if they so desire.

DEPRESSION CASE STUDY

*D*ebra is a 54-year-old woman with no significant mental health history. She recently saw her family physician for vague complaints of fatigue, restlessness, and insomnia, which she felt were attributed to "going through the change." Debra's menstrual cycles became irregular then ceased entirely 1 year ago. Her physician recommended light exercise and a hormone replacement medication. One week later, Debra's husband noted that she no longer had any desire to go with him to flea markets (a favorite weekend activity) and she seemed listless and apathetic. Her sleep problems worsened and she found herself waking at 2:00-3:00 a.m. and unable to return to sleep. Her appetite started to decrease and she frequently "forgot" to make the family's evening meal as she usually did complaining of exhaustion. Debra started experiencing intense headaches nearly every day causing her to always keep the curtains drawn and the lights low. Her symptoms exacerbated rapidly following the death of her favorite cat due to old age. She began crying uncontrollably, even at supermarkets, and refused to go out in public anymore. Her husband noticed that she was in the house either pacing in an agitated, purposeless manner or she was staring off into space; even television could no longer distract her. Over the course of a month, she lost 15 lb from her 145-lb frame. She started to talk to her husband about "the hereafter" and what to do with her possessions "once I am gone". He insisted she see a therapist who immediately referred Debra for an evaluation with a psychiatric Clinical Nurse Specialist. The CNS took a thorough history to rule out any concomitant illnesses or drug/alcohol abuse, and ordered some baseline lab tests including a thyroid panel. The lab tests showed only a mild dehydration, but were otherwise normal. The CNS then prescribed Lexapro® (escitalopram) 10 mg once daily for depression plus a p.r.n. of Restoril® (temazepam) 15 mg h.s. for the insomnia. The therapist continued to work with Debra and her husband educating them both as to the illness of depression. He also helped Debra to learn some cognitive strategies to deal with day-to-day stressors. Debra reported an improved mood and sleep within a week. By the fourth week her husband stated she was "nearly back to herself." At the end of 6 weeks, Debra felt "normal" again and was able to terminate therapy, but agreed to continue taking the antidepressant. She no longer needed the p.r.n. sleeping medication.

NURSING CARE PLAN

Problem Listing

- Fatigue
- Changes in ADLs
- Insomnia
- Hopelessness
- Dysmenorrhea
- Suicidal thoughts
- Weight loss
- Altered family relationships
- Crying episodes
- Poor concentration
- Impaired decision-making
- Socially isolating self

Priority Nursing Diagnosis

Self-care deficit related to persistent depressed mood as evidenced by fatigue, hopelessness, poor hygiene, and social isolation.

Long-term Goal

Client will return to her previous functioning level.

Short-term Objectives

1. Client will not remain in bed all day.

2. Client will resume previous activities with husband (e.g., flea markets) within 2 weeks.

3. Client will resume household responsibilities (e.g., cooking meals) within 2 weeks.

Nursing Interventions

1. Assist the client in making a daily living schedule and post this in a prominent place in the home.

2. Help the client and husband to identify places to go for diversional recreation no less than twice a week.

3. Provide medication education to the client and husband.

4. Assist the client in evaluating sleep patterns and develop a sleep hygiene plan (e.g., reduced caffeine, getting up at the same time every day, h.s. sedatives) to facilitate improved sleeping patterns.

5. Instruct the client to engage in 20-30 minutes of brisk walking daily (preferably outdoors if the weather is permitting).

6. Instruct the client in a healthy diet with plenty of fruits and vegetables. Daily multivitamins can be recommended.

7. Encourage the client to continue her regular church attendance.

CHAPTER 8
Questions 50-56

50. Significant symptoms of depression include

    a. mood changes, fatigue, sleep and appetite disturbances.

    b. euphoria, restlessness, and irrational spending sprees.

    c. agitation, confusion, and bizarre or unusual behaviors.

    d. paranoid delusions and reports of persistent hallucinations.

51. Dysthymia in adult clients is a depressive disorder characterized by

    a. chronic symptoms of depression lasting over 2 years.

    b. short-term depressive episodes lasting a few months.

    c. symptoms of suicidal ideation or self-injury.

    d. cyclic mood changes corresponding with the weather.

52. Postpartum depression usually occurs

    a. immediately after delivery.

    b. 1 week after delivery.

    c. in the first 4 weeks after delivery.

    d. several months after delivery.

53. Cognitive behavior therapy techniques offer distinct advantages to clients because

    a. insurance companies reimburse at a better rate.

    b. clients are taught to challenge beliefs that are detrimental to recovery.

    c. childhood traumas are thoroughly explored.

    d. of the use of positive and negative reinforcers.

54. ECT is utilized primarily to treat

    a. schizophrenia.

    b. treatment-resistant depression.

    c. severe aggression and agitation.

    d. epilepsy.

55. Tricyclic antidepressants

    a. are the current medications of choice in the treatment of depression.

    b. have few side effects.

    c. are not sedating.

    d. can cause serious cardiac arrhythmias.

56. Selective serotonin reuptake inhibitors

    a. have numerous dangerous side effects.

    b. are the current pharmacological treatment of choice.

    c. can cause significant cardiac arrhythmias.

    d. have a high risk for drug-food interactions.

CHAPTER 9

BIPOLAR SPECTRUM DISORDERS

CHAPTER OBJECTIVE

At the end of this chapter the reader will be able to identify symptoms of bipolar spectrum disorders and discuss appropriate nursing care and medication treatment.

LEARNING OBJECTIVES

At the end of this chapter, the reader will be able to

1. differentiate the symptoms of bipolar I and bipolar II disorders.

2. compare symptoms of an adult bipolar disorder from childhood bipolar disorders.

3. discuss mood stabilizing medications and their side effects.

4. describe nursing interventions for the client with mania.

BIPOLAR SPECTRUM DISORDERS

Bipolar disorders have been recognized since Emile Kraepelin first developed his classification and labeling system in the late 1800s. Descriptions of elevated and expansive moods alternating with periods of sluggishness or lethargy were described, along with stationary or "fundamental" non-impairing baseline states. Kraepelin called these disorders "manic-depressive," a term that persisted until the *DSM-IV* revision in 1994 when the name was changed to "bipolar" (Manning, 2002). The prevalence of bipolar spectrum disorders are between 1% and 5% in the general population. Bipolar II disorder has not been well described and there may be actually more cases than previously recognized. Depression is often the presenting symptom in bipolar II disorder, with diagnosing delays of up to 12 years, and a history of three to four different psychiatric consultations before the disorder is recognized (Manning, 2002). Bipolar I disorder is more clearly recognizable as the symptom presentation is often overt mania that may or may not be associated with psychosis. Bipolar spectrum disorders have a familial association, 5-24% for bipolar I and 1-5% for bipolar II, suggesting a genetic component to these disorders. The causes for bipolar spectrum disorders are unclear but they are believed to be related to an imbalance of chemicals in the brain called neurotransmitters. To diagnose a bipolar disorder, the client must demonstrate either manic, hypomanic or mixed manic/depressive moods between periods of depression.

Mania

1. The individual must have a period of abnormal and elevated, expansive, or irritable mood lasting at least 1 week (or less if hospitalization is required).

2. Three or more of the following symptoms must be present (four if the mood is predominantly depressed):

   a. inflated self-esteem or grandiosity.

   b. reduced need for sleep (3-4 hours or even none at all for days).

   c. pressured speech or talkativeness.

   d. racing thoughts or flight-of-ideas.

   e. distractibility.

   f. increased activity (either goal-directed or purposeless).

   g. high-risk behaviors (e.g., sexual indiscretions, spending sprees, bizarre business investments).

The manic symptoms must be significant to cause impairment in functioning (social relationships, work situations, or school settings). Manic symptoms also may not be associated with substance abuse (e.g., amphetamines or cocaine), a general medical condition (e.g., hyperthyroidism, adrenal gland tumor), or with medications (e.g., corticosteroids, antimalarials).

Women with postpartum-onset mania report depression during pregnancy up to 50% of the time (Kruger & Braunig, 2002). Psychotic symptoms can develop within 48-72 hours and are particularly dangerous for the mother and child.

Hypomania

The symptoms of hypomania are essentially the same as for mania, but to a lesser degree. The client must have a period of persistently elevated, expansive, or irritable moods that last at least 4 days, and that is a distinct change from baseline moods and behavior. Three or more of the criterion-2 symptoms must be present (four if the mood is predominantly irritable). The changes in moods and behaviors have to be easily recognized by others, but they cannot be severe enough to warrant hospitalization. Psychotic symptoms do not occur with hypomania; if psychosis is seen, then the diagnosis must be bipolar I disorder.

Mixed

Mixed manic/depressive symptoms have to be present for at least 1 week. Criteria for both mania and major depression are met nearly every day during this period. Individuals may demonstrate rapidly alternating mood shifts (anger, euphoria, sadness), agitation, insomnia, appetite problems, psychotic symptoms, or suicidal thoughts. Suicide attempts are high in this population due to the high level of distress felt by the client (as opposed to both mania and hypomania where clients generally feel little distress, but others report significant problems with the erratic behaviors). Mixed presentations are more common in children and adolescents.

BIPOLAR I DISORDER

A bipolar I disorder is diagnosed when a client experiences one or more clearly manic or mixed manic/depressive episodes. Often the client has had a history of depression that has chiefly resolved. Bipolar I disorder is cyclical; manic states will be alternated with periods of normal functioning and episodes of depression. These cycles are not necessarily proportionate as clients may experience two to three manic episodes for every single depressed state, nor are the cycles always predictable. Some individuals may cycle regularly every 6 months (usually in the fall and the spring), but in others no clear pattern can be distinguished. Psychotic symptoms may occur that are usually characterized by delusions of grandeur, paranoid delusions, ideas of reference, or auditory hallucinations. Individuals with bipolar I disorder can be significantly disabled by the condition, or they may be highly functional and hold esteemed positions in fields such as law, medicine, or business.

BIPOLAR II DISORDER

Bipolar II disorder is characterized by the occurrence of one or more significant depressive episodes, alternated with hypomania at least once. Hypomania is most likely to occur immediately following an episode of depression. Clients with bipolar II disorder may have difficulty in differentiating hypomania from "feeling good"; often the sleep disturbance associated with hypomania is the clue. Reports from family members of significant others will help to establish the diagnosis. Clients with bipolar II disorder who are treated solely with antidepressants may report difficulties in remaining at baseline.

CYCLOTHYMIC DISORDER

Clients with cyclothymic disorder present with a history of chronic, fluctuating moods with numerous periods of hypomanic and depressed symptoms, none of which require hospitalization, reach the point of psychosis, or meet the criteria for major depression. Cyclothymic disorder persists for at least 2 years or more (1 year in children and adolescents) and the client may be described by others as moody, unpredictable, or temperamental.

BIPOLAR DISORDER IN CHILDHOOD

Children with bipolar disorders almost always have a mixed presentation. Cycling of moods is less clear than in adult clients, and the presentation of mania may be less euphoric and more agitated, with explosive anger outbursts and violent episodes occurring. These outbursts can be triggered with little provocation (e.g., *"No. You can't have another cookie."*), and both the degree of the outburst and its duration may be extremely frightening for those around the child. Temper tantrums in children are usually self-limiting and respond to firm directives (*"Go to your room now!"*). Outbursts seen in a child with a bipolar disorder are much more intense and may involve hitting or kicking adults (including schoolteachers or administrators), attempting to bite, throwing things, destroying property, attacking pets or younger children, or using weapons (such as a dinner fork) against others. The duration of these episodes can last from 30 minutes to several hours and they usually don't end until the child exhausts himself. Children with this type of behavior are often diagnosed as "bipolar disorder, not otherwise specified", or "mood disorder, bipolar type." Bipolar disorders are strongly associated with attention deficit/hyperactivity disorder of childhood.

"Classic" bipolar I disorder is also seen in childhood. The presentation of bipolar I disorder in a child is similar to an adult's with pronounced sleep problems and an elevated or expansive mood accompanied by either euphoria or irritability. Children with bipolar I disorder commonly also experience some psychotic symptoms including delusions of grandeur (*"I'm Spiderman and I can shoot webs out of my hands!"*), or hallucinations (*"Grandpa came as an angel to my room to talk to me last night."*)

TREATMENT INTERVENTIONS

Management of a client with a bipolar spectrum disorder must be responsive to the state experienced by the client at that point in time. During episodes of major depression, the client may need activity of daily living (ADL) support, cognitive behavior or supportive therapy, and monitoring of nutrition or physical health (review Chapter 8: Major Depression and Related Disorders). During manic or hypomanic phases, staff may have to be firm and set limits on inappropriate behaviors. Clients in the throes of a full-blown mania are usually hospitalized for their own protection (to prevent them from carrying out fantastic plans or behaving bizarrely in the community), or for the protection of others (to prevent direct or indirect harm to others due to irrational or delusional beliefs of the client). The ethical issue of liberty versus respect for the client arises as a health care provider makes difficult decisions when caring for an overtly manic client. Manic clients are also unpredictable; assaultive behavior can occur rapidly and without apparent provocation. Families may not understand the illogical thoughts and actions by the client, and they can experience feelings of anger, disbelief or denial. Clients with hypomania are highly productive in the workplace or at home. Clients with mania are at risk for losing their employment because of their symptoms; clients often need to be encouraged to take a medical

leave-of-absence until their symptoms are remitted. During baseline states, education is paramount for both the client and family. Understanding mania, hypomania, and mixed symptoms as a psychiatric disorder will help the family to avoid feeling hurt or betrayed when the client "cycles" again. Helping the client to develop an increased awareness of the specific symptomatology (which is often consistent for each episode of mania/hypomania) will help to manage the disorder more effectively. Clients should also be instructed that insight is frequently lacking during hypomanic/manic cycles, and that they may have to trust others, rely on their opinions, and follow their advice when manic symptoms are developing.

TABLE 9-1: MEDICATIONS FOR MOOD STABILIZATION IN BIPOLAR SPECTRUM DISORDERS

Category	Generic Name	Trade Name	Sedation	Weight Gain	Hepatic Risk	Renal Risk	Risk for Blood Dyscrasias	Serum Monitoring Recommended	Comments
Lithium	lithium carbonate lithium citrate	Eskalith CR® Lithobid®	+	++	—	+++	—	Lithium levels, BUN, Creatinine, TSH	Closely bound with sodium Dehydration may cause toxicity Risk for hypothyroidism
Antiepileptics	divalproex	Depakote® Depakote ER®	+++ ++	++ ++	+++ +++	— —	+ +	VAL, SGOT, SGPT, CBC	Liver problems in very young children
	valproic acid	Depakene®	+++	++	+++	—	+	VAL, SGOT, SGPT, CBC	Very high in GI irritation so rarely prescribed
	carbamazepine	Tegretol®	++	+	—	—	+++	Carbamazepine level, CBC	Risk for ↓ WBC Risk for Stevens-Johnson rash
	oxcarbazepine	Trileptal®	++	+	—	—	—	—	No WBC issues; good in bipolar disorder II
	topiramate	Topamax®	+	—	—	—	—	—	Weight loss, slow titration avoids cognitive clouding
	gabapentin	Neurontin®	+++	—	—	—	—	—	Useful in chronic pain & bipolar disorder II
	lamotrigine	Lamictal®	++	+	—	—	—	—	Watch for Stevens-Johnson rash
	tiagabine	Gabitril®	+++	—	—	—	—	—	Sedating, benzodiazepine-like
Antipsychotics	olanzapine	Zyprexa®	+++	+++	+	—	—	Glucose, cholesterol	Only antipsychotic approved as a mood stabilizer; weight gain ↑
	risperidone	Risperdal®	++	++	+	—	—	Prolactin	Commonly used in children
	quetiapine	Seroquel®	+++	++	+	—	—	—	Sedating; less effective in bipolar disorder
	ziprasidone	Geodon®	+	—	+	—	—	—	Induces hypomania in low doses
	aripiprazole	Abilify™	++	—	+	—	—	—	No data yet; looks useful
	clozapine	Clozaril®	+++	+++	++	—	+++	WBC biweekly	Some data in schizoaffective disorder
Benzodiazepine	clonazepam	Klonopin®	++	—	+	—	—	—	Habit-forming/dependence

+++ High   ++ Moderate   + Low   — Negligible

MEDICATION INTERVENTIONS

Antidepressants

Antidepressants are utilized during the major depression component of a bipolar I or II disorder. Tricyclic antidepressants (TCAs) and selective serotonin reuptake inhibitors (SSRIs) are powerful mania-inducers when used in the absence of a mood stabilizer in a bipolar client. Buproprion (Wellbutrin SR®) is often preferred because of its prominent dopamine activity. Bipolar disorder (particularly type II) frequently does not get diagnosed until after a client has been exposed to antidepressants and the client rapidly develops hypomanic or full-blown manic symptoms. Client education with antidepressant medications needs to always include informing the client and family of this possibility. Mood stabilizers are necessary to prevent or reduce the occurrence and intensity of manic symptoms. An overview of mood stabilizing medications is provided in Table 9-1, and a discussion of these follows.

Lithium

Lithium was first discovered in 1817, when it was touted as a cure for gout and epilepsy. In 1949, it was first utilized in the treatment of manic/depressive symptoms in clients in Australia, but it was not available in the United States until 1970, due to the deaths of two cardiac patients who received lithium chloride as a salt substitute. Lithium is not patentable as it is a naturally occurring element, similar to sodium (Keltner et al., 2003). Brand names of lithium include Eskalith® and Lithonate®, both of which are extended release formulations. Lithium has traditionally been the treatment of choice for the bipolar client since the 1970s. It is effective predominantly for mania states, and can be helpful as an adjunctive treatment to antidepressants. Lithium is a naturally occurring mineral that displaces sodium at the cell membrane, but how this treats and prevents mania

is unknown. It is well absorbed orally and primarily excreted via the kidneys. Lithium has a narrow therapeutic versus toxic range. Serum monitoring is required when initiating this drug and annually thereafter. Lithium competes with antidiuretic hormone (ADH) in the renal collecting tubules and can precipitate diabetes insipidus. A significant number of clients on lithium maintenance treatment will develop hypothyroidism. Additionally, lithium toxicity has been associated with permanent renal insufficiency (Manning, 2002). Common side effects of lithium, even at therapeutic levels, include nausea, diarrhea, tremor, weight gain, polyuria, mild drowsiness, and a perception of cognitive dulling. Some clients may also have problems with fluid retention. Lithium toxicity most frequently occurs when the balance of fluids and electrolytes (particularly sodium) become abnormal and dehydration results. Excessive diarrhea or vomiting, sweating, or the use of diuretics (e.g., Lasix®, Dyazide®) can all precipitate lithium toxicity. Clients who are lithium toxic will display worsened diarrhea and vomiting, ataxia (staggering gait), restlessness, confusion, and agitation. Emergency care is indicated to avoid renal failure. Clients taking lithium may also experience a polygenic polydipsia (excess and unquenchable thirst) that can cause so much free fluid to be taken in that both sodium and potassium levels drop dangerously resulting in cardiac arrhythmias. Fluid restrictions in a hospital setting are the treatment for this disorder. Lithium is contraindicated in cardiac disease, and in pregnancy due to an increased risk for fetal heart defects.

Antiepileptics

Lithium is used less frequently today than are antiepileptics in the treatment of bipolar disorder. In general, the antiepileptic drugs are better tolerated and safer than lithium with similar treatment efficacy. Medications currently being prescribed include Depakote®, Depakote ER®, Tegretol®,

Trileptal®, Topamax®, Neurontin®, and Lamictal®. Phenytoin (Dilantin®) is an antiepileptic that does not have any positive treatment effects for bipolar disorder; in fact it is associated with irritability and anger problems.

Divalproex/valproic acid (Depakote®, Depakote ER®, Depakene®) has been used since the 1960s to treat epilepsy. During the course of its use, it was noted to have a calming effect in clients. The U.S. Food and Drug Administration (FDA) approved it for use as a primary agent for bipolar disorder in the late 1990s. It is generally well tolerated by the client. Valproic acid (Depakene®) has more problems with gastrointestinal (GI) upset than does divalproex (Depakote®, Depakote ER®) so it is rarely prescribed. Common side effects include nausea, diarrhea, sedation, weight gain, tremor, and hair loss. Multivitamins plus chromium are sometimes recommended when clients notice hair thinning. Elevations in liver enzymes can occur. Pancreatitis and liver failure have been associated with divalproex/valproic acid especially in young children. Toxicity can occur at serum levels higher than 125 ng/ml indicated by ataxia, confusion, slurred speech, and delirium. Serum monitoring of liver function enzymes is recommended at baseline, when a therapeutic dose is achieved, and annually thereafter. Divalproex dosage can be determined through serum level checks as well. Depakote ER® is also approved for migraine headache prevention at low, once-daily doses. Additionally, Depakote® and Depakote ER® have been utilized for agitation and aggression in the dementia population with good results. Divalproex and valproic acid are teratogenic and should not be used during pregnancy due to an increased risk of neural tube defects such as spina bifida.

Carbamazepine (Tegretol®) has been shown to be effective in bipolar I disorder as well. While it is generally well tolerated, side effects include nausea, sedation, drowsiness, and occasional loss or appetite. The significant risk for agranulocytosis in clients taking Tegretol® requires that serum monitoring of white blood counts (WBC)/complete blood counts (CBCs) be done initially when a therapeutic dose is reached, and annually thereafter. Any signs of cold or infection in a client taking Tegretol® should prompt an immediate CBC check. If blood dyscrasias do occur, the medication must be stopped. A new medication related to Tegretol® is oxcarbazepine (Trileptal®). Trileptal® can have the same GI and sedation side effects of Tegretol®, but it does not appear to cause any drops in WBCs or other blood changes. Serum testing is not recommended for Trileptal®. It may be more effective for bipolar II disorder than bipolar I, but its use is still fairly early in the mental health setting.

Topiramate (Topamax®) is gaining increasing popularity due to its anorectic side effects. Overweight clients have reported significant weight losses when adding Topamax® to their other medications as an adjunctive treatment. Topamax® has not been well studied as a single agent for bipolar disorder. Its side effects are relatively low with some complaints of dizziness and GI distress. Topamax® is mildly activating; some clients may report insomnia, anxiety, or restlessness. The most significant problem with utilizing Topamax® is the necessity for gradual titration due to problems with cognitive clouding or dulling. Serum level monitoring is not recommended for Topamax®.

Gabapentin (Neurontin®) is an interesting antiepileptic that has treatment efficacy for Bipolar disorder (primarily type II), as well as chronic pain conditions and peripheral neuropathies. Neurontin® has some activity on the anxiety-related neurotransmitter gamma amino-butyric acid (GABA), which also gives it anxiolytic properties as well. Neurontin is well tolerated with side effects of dizziness and sedation. Titration is usually required to avoid excessive fatigue or staggering gaits. Serum level monitoring is not necessary with this product.

Lamotrigine (Lamictal®) has shown treatment efficacy in rapid cycling and mixed mood states of bipolar disorder. Side effects of Lamictal® include insomnia, jitteriness, headache, and a mild reduction in appetite. Concerns over a progressive, excoriating rash known as Stevens-Johnson syndrome have led clinicians to use caution with Lamictal®, so it is not currently prescribed commonly in the mental health setting.

New Generation Antipsychotics

The newer generation antipsychotics (Clozaril®, Risperdal®, Zyprexa®, Seroquel®, Geodon®, and Abilify™) all demonstrate some antimanic properties (these medications are covered more thoroughly in Chapter 4: Schizophrenia and Related Disorders). Of these, only Zyprexa® has received FDA approval for its use as a primary agent in bipolar disorder. Serum levels are not necessary with these antipsychotic medications as their potential for toxicity is low. Pregnancy studies have not been completed, but there is no clear evidence of fetal toxicity (as seen with lithium and valproic acid).

Zyprexa® rapidly reduces the agitation and increased motor activity seen in manic clients, and it stabilizes moods for ongoing use. Side effects of Zyprexa® include sedation, occasionally restlessness, and increased appetite. Weight gains associated with Zyprexa® have been pronounced with up to 50 lb reported by adult clients, and 20 lb seen in children. Not all clients will gain weight, however, so the medication should not be avoided for this reason alone.

Clozaril® (clozapine) has several small studies indicating its efficacy in schizoaffective disorders (Dittman, Forsthoff, Thoma, & Grunze, 2002), but its use is limited by the FDA requirement for weekly WBC monitoring for the first 6 months of treatment, followed by biweekly thereafter for life. Other side effects of Clozaril® are salivation, sedation, and weight gain. A small percentage of clients taking Clozaril® develop seizure disorders over time.

Risperdal® is frequently utilized in child psychiatry as a mood stabilizing agent. It blocks dopamine release and seems to be effective in reducing agitation, anger outbursts, and the violent episodes seen in childhood-associated bipolar disorder with mixed mood presentations. Risperdal® is less effective for mood swings in adult clients. Children may require a dose that is only one-third that of an adult. This low dosing (<3mg/day) helps to minimize side effects that include tremors, weight gain, sedation, and a risk for extrapyramidal syndrome and tardive dyskinesia.

Quetiapine (Seroquel®) has one study that addressed its use in combination with Depakote® in treating bipolar disorder in adolescents (DelBello, Schwiers, Rosenberg, & Strakowski, 2002). Seroquel® in combination with Depakote® was found to be more effective for the treatment of bipolar mania in this population than was Depakote® alone. Side effects to Seroquel® include sedation, nausea, headache, and GI upset. Seroquel® is often used off-label as an adjunct to children with attention-deficit/hyperactivity disorder associated with insomnia and aggression.

Ziprasidone (Geodon®) yielded a greater improvement in manic symptoms as compared to a placebo in one study of 197 adults with mania (Perlis, Evins, Ogutha, & Sachs, 2002). Geodon® is an activating antipsychotic useful in the treatment of depression. Geodon® may precipitate hypomanic behaviors in low doses. It is recommended that Geodon® be dosed more rapidly and on the higher end of the dosing spectrum to avoid these symptoms. Early concerns with cardiac conduction delays have not been demonstrated in clinical practice. Some clinicians may prefer to obtain 12-lead electrocardiograms (EKGs) or avoid the use of this medication in a client with cardiac disease, but this is not required. Geodon® is available in a rapid-acting injectable dose that will soon replace the use of traditional antipsychotic injections (Haldol®, Thorazine®) in the emergency department.

Aripiprazole (Abilify™) was approved by the FDA in November of 2002 for the treatment of schizophrenia. Its use in bipolar disorder has not been investigated, although some clinicians are reporting positive benefits in antimanic properties. Abilify™ works gradually achieving its maximum therapeutic potential in about 4 weeks. Sedation is the predominant side effect reported.

Benzodiazepines

Benzodiazepines have potent antianxiety and antiepileptic properties. They are not used in epilepsy as primary agents because of problems with drug dependency, tolerance, and withdrawal. Short-acting agents (e.g., Ativan®) are quite useful in the emergency department for treating an agitated or manic client. Ativan® can be given orally, intramuscularly, or intravenously. Clonazepam (Klonopin®) is the best choice for maintenance care of the bipolar client as an adjunctive treatment to antiepileptic or antipsychotic agents. Klonopin® has a longer half-life with treatment effects lasting 12-16 hours. Its side effects include sedation, and dizziness or ataxia at higher doses. Klonopin® is a central nervous system (CNS) depressant, and its sedation effects will be potentiated by other CNS depressants, or medications metabolized by the enzyme cytochrome P450 such as Prozac®.

NURSING MANAGEMENT DURING MANIA

Nursing care of the manic client can be quite challenging. Protecting clients from inadvertently harming themselves or their reputations, and protecting others from being physically or emotionally harmed by the clients is foremost. Many manic clients require hospitalization and clear nursing behavior care plans. Manic clients have a ten-dency to be pushy, noisy, and intrusive, and to test their limits continuously. Staff members need to maintain clear lines of communication with one another to prevent staff-splitting behaviors by the client. The nurse also needs to adopt a caring but firm approach and provide external structure for the client in the form of established routines, rules, and consistent behavior consequences. Manic clients may forget to eat or to bathe. It is up to the nurse to see that the clients basic needs are taken care of. It may be necessary to limit telephone calls to give family members a rest from constant demands by the client. Clients with mania suffer from distractibility and a loss of control. Reducing environmental stimuli by providing private rooms, scheduling rest periods, allowing time for exercise, and limiting contact with other clients may be helpful. Insomnia is a major problem for manic clients. Administering at bedtime (h.s.) sedatives and as needed (p.r.n.) medications throughout the night, keeping lights and noise levels low, and requiring that the client remain in the room (not at the nurses station talking with staff or on the phone) during the night will be helpful. Staff should be cautious not to trigger aggression in a client who is manic. Impulse control is extremely poor, and even an apparently minor comment may cause the client to begin escalating. When signs of increasing tension are seen (pacing, clenched fists, raised voice, darting eye contact), the client should be offered a p.r.n. medication (usually a benzodiazepine) and asked to wait quietly in the room until the medicine has worked. Nursing staff that regularly work with manic clients should be well trained in seclusion and restraint policies and procedures, and have adequate staffing backup should it be necessary to utilize restraints (four to six persons).

BIPOLAR I DISORDER CASE STUDY

Pablo is a 22-year-old man who has completed 2 years of fine arts study in a major university. Always creative, he started to find himself unable to stop painting or sketching until well into the night. Eventually, he found himself able to stay up for more than 48 hours with little effort. His friends commented that he always seemed to be "on a natural high" and he was "fun to be around." Pablo was very productive in his painting, but he started to miss classes as he began to think that there was nothing they could teach him that he didn't already know. After a few weeks, Pablo's irregular hours and poor eating habits caused him to look thin and tired. His energy level became more frenetic and agitated, and his friends stopped visiting — now he seemed to be irritable and short-tempered, plus they were tired of hearing about his "genius talent." One day, when Pablo had been awake for 4 consecutive days, he called his parents to tell them about the "great opportunity" he would have if they would buy him a plane ticket to Paris. He was certain that the Louvre' would hang his paintings and give him a private showing on the spot, after all he felt he was "channeling the spirit and soul of Van Gogh." When his parents questioned this, Pablo became agitated saying he would get the money "somehow" and no one would stop him. Subsequently, Pablo was arrested for attempted robbery of a convenience store. The arresting officer put in his report that "the perpetrator was shouting obscenities and appeared to be talking to someone he kept calling 'Vince'." Pablo was admitted to a secure psychiatric facility on an immediate detention order. He initially required four-way restraints and chemical sedation. He was started on Depakote ER® (valproic acid) and titrated to 2,500 mg/day. Additionally, he was prescribed Zyprexa® at 20 mg at bedtime (q h.s.) and was given p.r.n. doses of Ativan® (lorazepam). After 7 days inpatient, he was discharged to his parents' home for further recuperation.

NURSING CARE PLAN

Problem Listing

- Altered mood states — agitation, excitability
- Altered thoughts — delusions of grandeur, ideas of reference, auditory hallucinations
- Inadequate sleep
- Poor nutrition
- Knowledge deficit regarding his illness or medications
- Potential for harm to self or others

Priority Nursing Diagnosis

Potential for harm to self or others related to altered thoughts (grandiosity, ideas of reference) as evidenced by extreme agitation and irrational behaviors.

Long-term Goal

Client will no longer demonstrate any evidence of psychosis.

Short-term Objectives

1. Client will not harm self during the hospital stay.

2. Client will not harm others (staff, visitors) during the hospital stay.

3. Client will demonstrate compliance with recommended medication treatment.

Nursing Interventions

1. Nurse will administer p.r.n. medications at the first sign of increasing agitation.

2. Nurse will educate the client in relaxation techniques to help in reducing anxiety.

3. Seclusion and restraints will be utilized by staff in a judicious manner and only when absolutely necessary.

4. Staff will adapt a nonconfrontational, supportive approach with client to minimize potential misperceptions due to altered thoughts.

5. Staff will keep the client in a private room until all risk for assaultive behavior has passed.

6. Staff may elect to restrict visitors if client's behavior is inappropriate.

EXAM QUESTIONS

CHAPTER 9
Questions 57-63

57. A bipolar I disorder has

    a. alternating episodes of depression with mania that may be accompanied by psychosis.

    b. consistently manic and baseline episodes with no history of depression.

    c. consistently depressed episodes alternated with periods of hypomania.

    d. chronically hypomanic and depressed episodes that last over 2 years.

58. A bipolar II disorder has

    a. alternating episodes of depression with mania that may be accompanied by psychosis.

    b. consistently manic and baseline episodes with no history of depression.

    c. consistently depressed episodes alternated with periods of hypomania.

    d. chronically depressed episodes that last over 2 years.

59. Bipolar disorder, not otherwise specified, in childhood can be expressed as

    a. occasional temper tantrums requiring time-outs.

    b. frequent explosive and violent anger outbursts.

    c. poor focus, decreased attention span, and an inability to concentrate.

    d. problems achieving developmental milestones.

60. Medications necessary to prevent or reduce mood swings are called

    a. sedative/hypnotics.

    b. antidepressants.

    c. antiepileptics.

    d. mood stabilizers.

61. The only antipsychotic approved for use as a primary mood stabilizer is

    a. Geodon®.

    b. Risperdal®.

    c. Clozaril®.

    d. Zyprexa®.

62. Manic clients can benefit from

    a. many visitors to provide distractions.

    b. reduced environmental stimulation and distractions.

    c. unrestricted access to telephone use.

    d. being permitted to skip therapeutic groups.

63. Symptoms that tell the nurse that a manic client is escalating and may need a p.r.n. medication include

    a. remaining socially isolated and refusing to participate in activities.

    b. shouting insults, cursing and slamming down the telephone.

    c. calling the physician names and threatening to sue the facility.

    d. pacing, clenched fists, a raised voice, and darting eye contact.

CHAPTER 10

ANXIETY DISORDERS

CHAPTER OBJECTIVE

At the end of this chapter the reader will be able to identify symptoms of an anxiety disorder and discuss relevant treatment including therapy and medications.

LEARNING OBJECTIVES

At the end of this chapter, the reader will be able to

1. describe the symptoms of anxiety.

2. differentiate generalized anxiety from other types of anxiety disorders.

3. discuss treatment for anxiety disorders including therapy and medications.

ANXIETY

Anxiety is a healthy, adaptive response that has a protective function in preventing an individual from harm. Anxiety stops us from engaging in high-risk activities and it helps us to think more clearly in emergency situations. It is only when anxiety becomes maladaptive that it becomes a problem. Hans Selye (1956) recognized that human beings respond to stress in characteristic ways regardless of the stressor experienced. He classified these changes into three distinct stages that he called the "General Adaptation Syndrome: Alarm, Resistance, and Exhaustion" (Keltner,

Schwecke, & Bostrom, 2003). In the alarm stage, a client develops a heightened awareness of the stressor and mobilizes resources to cope with it. Clear biological changes occur in the body to prepare the person for "fight or flight." These changes include discharges of norepinephrine and epinephrine, increased thyroid hormone and corticosteroid levels, a release of endogenous opiates, and diversion of blood from the organs to the skeletal muscles. During an alarm response, clients perceive an increased level of anxiety and other changes that are designed to prepare the person to deal with the stressor. Table 10-1 provides an overview of anxiety responses at the mild, moderate, severe, and panic levels and associates these with emotional, cognitive, and behavioral experiences of the client. If the stressor continues without resolution, the client will move into the next stage of resistance. During the resistance stage, the use of coping and defense mechanisms begin (Chapter 8) and physical symptoms may begin to develop. Chronically elevated epinephrine levels can lead to hypertension. Corticosteroids and gastric secretions are irritating to the gastric lining and may lead to ulcers or colitis. Headaches are common complaints, as are muscle aches or tension (particularly in the neck and back) and chronic pain. The third stage, called exhaustion, occurs when stressors persist over a long period of time and the client loses the ability to cope utilizing normal mechanisms. Thinking becomes illogical. Sensory misperceptions may

TABLE 10-1: OVERVIEW OF LEVELS OF ANXIETY

Level of Anxiety	Physical and Behavioral Changes	Emotional Changes	Cognitive Changes
Mild	Increased heart rate, BP Muscle tension Pupil dilation Frequent urination Blood shunts to skeletal muscles	Excitement Mild fear	Increased alertness Improved concentration Increased awareness of surroundings
Moderate	Further increases in heart rate, BP Need to pace; feelings of restlessness Body aches, muscle aches	Sense of foreboding (something about to happen)	Racing thoughts Trouble staying focused
Severe	Increased respiratory rates; hyperventilation Tremors, especially in hands GI upset: nausea, vomiting GI pain and diarrhea	Fearful, anxious or "nervous", sense of dread	Flight-of-ideas Inability to focus or concentrate Inability to listen well to others Decreased decision-making abilities
Panic	Wildly erratic vital signs Attempts to run away or flee Aggression or striking out Whole body tremors Suicidal/self-injury Immobilization	Overt fears: fear of dying, fear of injury	Irrationality Illogical thoughts Disorganized May be delusional

occur. Clients may become suicidal or violent, or they may shut down completely. Chronic and persistent anxiety early in life may lead to personality disorders or other dysfunctional ways of dealing with life later on. Exhaustion is a contributing factor to Battered Women's Syndrome and domestic violence (covered more thoroughly in Chapter 12).

The *DSM-IV-TR* recognizes and describes over 12 different types of anxiety disorders. For the purposes of this book, the following disorders will be reviewed: generalized anxiety disorder, panic disorder (with and without agoraphobia), social anxiety disorder, specific phobias, posttraumatic stress disorder, obsessive-compulsive disorder, and pediatric autoimmune neuropsychiatric disorder associated with group A Streptococci (PANDAS).

GENERALIZED ANXIETY DISORDER

A generalized anxiety disorder (GAD) occurs when a person experiences chronic and persistent anxiety, without a specific focus or cause,

over a period of at least 6 months. Associated with muscle tension, there may be problems with trembling, feeling shaky inside, and muscle aches or soreness. Sweating, nausea, and diarrhea are common and an exaggerated startle response may occur. Children with GAD tend to be overly perfectionistic about the quality of their schoolwork and they worry about criticism from teachers or other authority figures. They may have excessive concerns about punctuality or worry about catastrophic events, or adult responsibilities such as paying the bills. They seek out constant reassurance from others, and they may complain of vague stomachaches or headaches. *DSM-IV-TR* criteria for diagnosing GAD include the following:

1. Excessive anxiety and worry more days than not for at least 6 months about a number of different things

2. The client finds it difficult to control the worry

3. Three or more of the following symptoms are present (only one is required in children):

   a. restlessness or feeling keyed up or on edge

b.   easily fatigued

c.   difficulty concentrating

d.   irritability

e.   muscle tension

f.   sleep disturbance (usually delayed onset or restlessness)

To meet the criteria for GAD, there cannot be a specific focus or worry such as seen in phobic disorders, or clear cause as identified in posttraumatic stress disorder, and the symptoms must significantly interfere with functioning in the community.

Therapy for GAD

Cognitive behavior therapy, supportive therapy, and even psychoanalysis are all helpful in treating GAD. Learned patterns from childhood may have a significant impact on the development of the disorder. For example, a child who is bullied and threatened by siblings, and criticized by parents, may grow into an adult who is always tensed up and waiting for someone to bully, intimidate, or criticize. This can become a self-fulfilling prophecy if that person chooses a spouse or employer who is domineering or abusive. Counseling can help a client to uncover some of the coping techniques, defense mechanisms, and learned beliefs. Hopefully change can occur as a result of improved awareness and insight. The therapist will also need to teach new tools and coping strategies to compensate for losing the more dysfunctional ones.

Relaxation Techniques and Guided Imagery

Educating the client in relaxation breathing and guided imagery is useful for reducing anxiety levels from severe or panic states to mild or moderate ones. During guided imagery, the client is asked to imagine a calm, peaceful, and safe place: What can be seen there? Smelled? Heard? Who else might be there? When the client is able to imagine being in a safe place, then they can be taught to allow fears to enter in and be confronted or thrown away.

Relaxation breathing is a systematic exercise of alternatively tensing and relaxing muscles in association with slow deep breaths until the sensation of tension is drained away. Relaxation breathing and guided imagery can be rehearsed in the office setting, and then utilized in any number of other settings when tension is building.

Exercise

The importance of exercise in treating GAD cannot be overemphasized. The physiological responses associated with anxiety prepare the body for "fight or flight." Physical exertion (difficult enough to cause an increase in heart rate and mild shortness of breath) will "trick" the body into believing that the survival response was initiated, therefore leading to a draining away of tension and anxiety. Exercise can range from a brisk walk to a jog, to weight lifting or a martial arts classes. Exercise "prescriptions" should be tailored to the client and take into consideration any pre-existing medical conditions.

MEDICATION INTERVENTIONS FOR ANXIETY

Four categories of medications are commonly prescribed for treating GAD: benzodiazepines, nonbenzodiazepine anxiolytics, antidepressants, and antihistamines. Other medications may be given including antiepileptics (e.g., Neurontin®) or new-generation antipsychotics (e.g., Seroquel®), but their use is less frequent and usually occurs only after other means have been tried. Of the medications available, current practice is to utilize selective serotonin reuptake inhibitors (SSRIs) as first-line treatment for all anxiety disorders, and supplement them with other agents as necessary.

All of the SSRIs are highly effective in treating anxiety. Paxil® has been approved specifically for panic disorder as well as depression. Zoloft® has been studied and received U.S. Food and Drug Administration (FDA) approval in both posttraumatic stress disorder and social anxiety/phobia disorder. Luvox® has a specific indication for obsessive compulsive disorder. The relationship between serotonin, norepinephrine, and anxiety symptoms is pronounced and these medications are clearly superior in reducing the overall experience of anxiety. Tricyclic antidepressants (TCAs) have also been used quite effectively in treating anxiety for years, but their use is limited by their extensive side effect profile and cardiac conduction problems. Anafranil® is a TCA that is approved specifically for the treatment of obsessive compulsive disorders. A detailed discussion of both SSRIs and TCAs is provided in Chapter 8.

Benzodiazepines are medications that work by enhancing the effects of the neurotransmitter gamma-aminobutyric acid (GABA). The action of GABA is to open chloride channels at the cellular level in the brain, which makes a neuron less responsive to other neurotransmitters, such as serotonin, norepinephrine, and dopamine. The overall effect is a slowing down of neuron firing. Benzodiazepines contribute to this brain-inhibition effect and slow down excitability, agitation, nervousness, and (often) alertness, attention span, concentration, and decision-making abilities. Some clients experience a paradoxical reaction to benzodiazepines (particularly Valium® and Librium®) and may become more agitated instead of less. Different types of benzodiazepines are covered more thoroughly in Chapter 6. Medications most commonly used include Xanax®, Ativan®, Valium®, and Klonopin®. Benzodiazepines have the distinct disadvantage of being habituating; tolerance quickly develops and more of the drug is needed to achieve the desired effect. When the client runs out of medications, withdrawal symptoms occur. Withdrawal to benzodiazepines is characterized by anxiety, restlessness, and panic attacks. The longer acting agents (Klonopin® and Valium®) are not as

difficult to manage as the shorter-acting ones (Xanax® and Ativan®). Withdrawal symptoms can develop within 8 hours of the last dose of Xanax® and 12 hours with Ativan®. A client who takes Xanax® three to four times a day (t.i.d.-q.i.d.) long enough to develop habituation (1-2 weeks), will wake up feeling anxious and in panic simply because of medication withdrawal effects.

Two nonbenzodiazepine anxiolytic medications are available for use in anxiety disorders. Buspirone (Buspar®) acts as a serotonin enhancer in the brain and has no activity on GABA. Buspar® is mildly sedating but it has no addictive properties so habituation is not an issue. Unfortunately, Buspar® can take 2-4 weeks or longer to be fully effective, and most clients want anxiety relief more rapidly (benzodiazepines are effective within 30 minutes or less following a single dose). Buspar® dosing is usually t.i.d.-q.i.d. as well, making it less convenient. Off-label uses for Buspar® have been used in treating impulsivity in developmentally delayed clients or individuals with dementia, and in treating hot flashes associated with natural or surgically-induced menopause. A second medication that is gaining more attention recently for its anxiolytic properties is tiagabine (Gabitril®). Gabitril® is another antiepileptic agent that seems to mimic or enhance the activity of a subtype of GABA. Gabitril® is not a benzodiazepine and it has no addictive properties. Some clients report significant anxiety relief with Gabitril®, although it tends to be activating in other clients causing them to feel restless or agitated. Gabitril® may also have some usefulness in bipolar disorders, particularly in bipolar II. Side effects to Gabitril® include dizziness, drowsiness, and unsteady gait.

Antihistamines can provide some assistance in the short-term treatment of anxiety. Antihistamines are added to preoperative medications (Vistaril®) to help reduce anxiety in the health care setting. Their anxiolytic properties are primarily through the side effect of sedation, which is perceived as calming to the client. Diphenhydramine (Benadryl®) is more useful in adults as many children may have a paradoxical reaction to it. Cyproheptadine (Periactin®) is an antihistamine with a mild serotonin activity that is helpful as an adjunct treatment for children with insomnia. Hydroxyzine (Vistaril®, Atarax®) is useful in adults and children as a calming agent or at bedtime (h.s.) sleep-enhancing medication. Antihistamines are relatively safe (Benadryl® is over-the-counter) and low in side effects.

PANIC DISORDER

Panic attacks can occur without warning. They consist of a discrete period of intense fear or discomfort in the absence of any real danger. The *DSM-IV-TR* criteria for a panic attack require four or more of the following symptoms:

1. palpitations, pounding heart, or increased heart rate
2. sweating
3. trembling or shaking
4. shortness of breath or "smothering" sensation
5. choking sensation
6. chest pain or tightness
7. nausea or abdominal distress
8. feeling dizzy, lightheaded, faint or unsteady
9. feelings of unreality or detachment
10. fear of losing control or going crazy
11. fear of dying
12. numbness or tingling sensations
13. chills or hot flushing

A panic attack may occur in association with another anxiety disorder, with major depression, or by itself. A trigger for the attack may or may not be apparent. Children may experience panic attack symptoms when asked to give a presentation in school, or when facing a fearful situation such as a blood draw (symptoms should however be differentiated from specific phobias such as a fear of needles). Clients usually present for initial treatment in an emergency department where they receive electrocardiogram (EKG) tracings, blood testing, and other services before being given sedatives and sent home. Panic disorder can be associated with suicide risk due to the intensity of the discomfort experienced. Panic attacks may occur once, weekly, monthly, or several times a day. They will usually persist from 30 minutes up to 4 hours at a time. A panic disorder develops when there is a presence of recurrent panic attacks followed by a persistent worry about having additional attacks, or a worry about the implications of the attack (e.g., losing control or "going crazy"), or when there is a significant change in the client's behavior related to the attacks. A fear of recurrent attacks may eventually cause the client to be afraid to leave the house, or be "caught" out in public. Agoraphobia occurs when the client changes behaviors to avoid situations where a panic attack might prove to be embarrassing, or from which escape may be difficult. For some clients, agoraphobia may be limited to an avoidance of long trips from home or extended bus rides. Other clients have more severe symptoms including the inability to leave one's own property or even to go outside of the house without having a panic attack or experiencing overwhelming anticipatory anxiety.

Panic disorder, with and without agoraphobia, is treated with a combination of exposure therapy and medications. Exposure therapy consists of supporting the client in making steps toward panic-inducing situations (e.g., going outside) while providing a great deal of reassurance and relaxation training. "Flooding" occurs when the client is thrust suddenly into a panic-inducing situation and not allowed to escape. "Flooding" can be emotionally traumatic, especially for a child, so its use is not routinely recommended. Panic symptoms can be alleviated by benzodiazepines, but they will do nothing to prevent reoccurrence. The best medical treatment for panic continues to be SSRI medications on a daily basis for adults and children. Benzodiazepines may be used as supplemental as needed (p.r.n.) drugs during panic-inducing situations. With treatment, panic symptoms may remit entirely or they may only be reduced to a more manageable level.

SOCIAL ANXIETY DISORDER

A social anxiety disorder is diagnosed when there is a persistent fear of social or performance situations in which humiliation or embarrassment may occur. Adults and most adolescents will recognize that their fear is unfounded (children typically do not have this level of cognitive awareness yet), but they are unable to prevent severe anxiety symptoms or panic attacks. Exposure to the social situation invariably provokes the anxiety (in children this may be expressed as immobilization ["freezing"], crying, tantrums, or shrinking away). Because of the anxiety symptoms, the client will make inordinate efforts to avoid the precipitant, which can range anywhere from isolated public speaking engagements, to a fear of all social situations (e.g., parties), to a fear of all places full of people (e.g., grocery store).

Treatment for social anxiety disorder consists of SSRI medications when the disorder is disabling to day-to-day living, and intermittent benzodiazepines when there is only rare exposure. Propanolol (Inderal®) is often prescribed for adult clients who must present research or perform in other public speaking venues. Inderal® decreases tremors and heart rate (elevations of which occur with moderate anxiety) and provides the clients with a sense that they are more in control. Inderal® does not produce the cognitive clouding and sense of mild euphoria as does a benzodiazepine (side effects to be avoided when speaking in front of a crowd). Nonmedical treatment consists of coaching

the clients to mentally rehearse the situation beforehand while imagining themselves as being charming, witty, and well-liked by the audience.

SPECIFIC PHOBIAS

The essential feature of a specific phobia is a persistent, intense, and irrational fear of a specific object, circumstance, or situation. Many types of specific phobias exist (agoraphobia, claustrophobia, hydrophobia) but they are all classified into five basic types

1. Animal type: fears are cued by animals (e.g., dogs, snakes) or by insects (e.g., spiders). Animal phobias typically have a childhood onset.

2. Natural environment type: fear is cued by natural occurrences, such as storms, lightning, tornadoes, or earthquakes. These disorders also frequently onset in childhood.

3. Blood-injection-injury type: fear is cued by seeing blood or an injury, or by receiving an injection or invasive procedure. This type is highly familial and is often accompanied by a vasovagal response (fainting).

4. Situational type: fear is cued by specific situations such as being in an airplane, a tunnel, a bridge, an elevator, enclosed places, or heights. This type tends to onset either in childhood, or in the mid-20s and is similar to a panic disorder.

5. Other type: fear is cued by any other stimuli which may include things such as a fear of choking or vomiting, a fear of contracting an illness, a fear of falling down; or children's fears of loud sounds or clowns.

Treatment of a specific phobia (if treatment is necessary) is to gradually expose the client to the feared object or situation after educating him or her to relaxation techniques and guided imagery. Exposure may start out with simply talking about the object or situation, then move on to looking at pictures (or drawing pictures), then to watching video and eventually to "field trips" for direct exposure. Medications are only necessary when exposure to the feared object or situation is unavoidable (e.g., airline travel), in which benzodiazepines are the best options. Children with severe-blood-injection-injury type may benefit from low doses of Ativan® prior to dental work or other necessary procedures (Valium® can produce paradoxical or manic-like reactions in young children).

POSTTRAUMATIC STRESS DISORDER

Posttraumatic stress disorder (PTSD) and acute stress disorder occur in response to an extreme stressor that involves personal experience of an event with actual or threatened death or serious injury; or witnessing an event that involves death or serious injury; or learning about unexpected or violent death, serious harm, or threat of death or injury to a family member or close friend. The client responds with feelings of intense fear, helplessness, or horror (children may express agitated or disorganized behaviors). In acute stress disorder, the symptoms from the trauma occur immediately and last from 2 days to 4 weeks. After this time period, the client may meet the criteria for PTSD. With an acute stress disorder, three or more of the following symptoms must be experienced to make the diagnosis:

1. a sense of numbing, detachment, or an absence of emotional responses

2. feeling dazed or unaware of one's surroundings

3. derealization (feeling as though in a dream)

4. depersonalization (feeling as though outside of oneself)

5. dissociative amnesia (can't remember parts or all of the trauma)

There must also be a persistent reexperience of the trauma through recurrent images dreams, thoughts, or flashbacks. Clients will avoid stimuli that arouse recollections of the trauma, and will exhibit symptoms of increased arousal states (insomnia, irritability, poor concentration, exaggerated startle, restlessness, and hypervigilance).

PTSD is more persistent and long lasting. It can occur immediately following the trauma, or memories can be repressed and symptoms occur years later. Clients with PTSD may describe guilty feelings about their experience (especially if others were injured or killed and they were not). Avoidance behaviors can lead to marital conflicts, work conflicts, or interpersonal problems. Severe cases may report auditory hallucinations or paranoia. Impulsive and self-destructive behaviors are associated with traumas related to physical or sexual abuse. Somatic complaints may be frequent. *DSM-IV-TR* criteria for PTSD are as follows:

1. The client was exposed to a traumatic event where

   a. there was actual or threatened death or serious injury or assault to the self or others; and

   b. the client's response involved intense fear, helplessness, or horror (agitated or disorganized behavior in children).

2. The traumatic event is persistently reexperienced in one or more of the following:

   a. recurrent memories of the event including images, thoughts or perceptions (children may reenact themes of the trauma through play)

   b. recurrent distressing dreams of the event (children may have vague, frightening dreams)

   c. feeling as if the event were reoccurring (e.g., flashbacks) (children may reenact portions of the event such as molesting younger children)

d. intense emotional distress in response to internal or external cues symbolic of the event

e. physical reactions to those internal or external cues

3. Persistent avoidance of anything related to the trauma, and a sense of numbing as indicated by three or more of the following:

a. avoids thoughts, feelings, or conversations related to the trauma

b. avoids activities, places, or people that arouse memories

c. unable to recall important aspects of the trauma

d. diminished interest in activities

e. feelings of detachment or estrangement

f. restricted range of affect

g. lack of a sense of a future

4. Persistent symptoms of increased arousal with two or more of the following:

a. difficulty falling or staying asleep

b. irritability or outbursts of anger

c. difficulty concentrating

d. hypervigilance (always "on guard")

e. exaggerated startle responses

5. Duration of the symptoms in criteria 2, 3, and 4 lasting more than 1 month

6. The disturbance causing clinically significant impairments in functioning

Treatment for acute stress disorder and PTSD usually involves intensive therapy. The therapist must first establish trust with the client. Psychoanalysis may be beneficial to help the client to uncover forgotten aspects of the trauma; a trained therapist may use hypnosis cautiously. For traumas that involve large groups of people (e.g., World Trade Center), it may be beneficial to set up small group discussions. When the client is ready, talking about the trauma is the first step to healing. Particularly horrendous experiences (such as ongoing childhood sexual abuse, or torture) may take years for the client to be able to discuss. Symptoms of anxiety, panic, and major depression will emerge as more memories are uncovered and discussed. Antidepressant medication use is usually beneficial — SSRIs are preferred for their low side-effect profiles and safety in overdosage. Assessing for suicidal or homicidal thoughts at different phases of recovery is essential. Alcohol and other substance abuse risk is high in individuals with acute stress disorder/PTSD. It may be helpful to provide education to the client as to "typical" responses that others experience following a trauma. This will serve to let clients know that they are not alone. Active listening and other therapeutic communication skills are more important than offering advice or expressing one's own opinions. Clients who have been traumatized need to be listened to, not lectured at.

OBSESSIVE-COMPULSIVE DISORDER

The essential characteristics of an obsessive-compulsive disorder (OCD) are recurrent obsessions (intrusive thoughts) or compulsions (ritualistic behaviors) that cause marked distress to the client, are usually unwanted, and are severe enough to be time consuming. The intrusive thoughts associated with obsessions may seem to come out of nowhere. They are not delusional in nature, because the client understands that they are irrational or illogical. Children with OCD may not recognize that their thoughts or actions are excessive or unreasonable. Common obsessions include fears of germ or disease contamination, repeated worry or doubt, a need to have things in order, sexual imagery, or occasionally aggressive or horrible acts. Individuals with obsessions initially attempt to ignore or suppress the thoughts, but almost always they will find behaviors that provide some temporary relief from the anxiety (defense mechanism of "undoing"). The compulsive behaviors may have some logical association with the obsession (e.g., washing hands with a germ fear, or praying over aggressive thoughts) or they may not. The most common compulsive behaviors include counting, checking, cleaning or washing, ordering, demanding assurances, or repeating actions. Panic attacks are associated with OCD when clients feel that they may not be able to carry out compulsions. Compulsive behaviors can take hours and be quite disabling for the client; for example, a client may feel the need to shower in a certain way every day and if the client deviates from the steps in any way, the client must start over at the beginning.

Consequences of OCD are impaired relationships with others, family and marital discord, and work or school conflicts, and possibly an inability to live life as fully and normally as possible. Skin conditions and infections can result in individuals with germ or contamination fears. OCD has a familial association and may have some genetic basis.

The most effective treatment for OCD is SSRI medications. The TCA Anafranil® (clomipramine) is also quite effective, but due to side effect risks the SSRIs should be first-line treatment. Luvox® is specifically indicated for OCD, but all of the medications in this class are effective. The miscellaneous category antidepressant Effexor XR® is highly effective as well. Wellbutrin SR® is less useful as it has prominent dopaminergic activity rather than serotonin. Exposure therapy is also indicated in treatment of OCD. For example, clients with a fear of contamination may be asked initially to simply touch a desktop or watch the therapist eat food off of the desktop, then progress to touching money, doorknobs, and eventually to shaking hands, all the while suppressing the compulsive urges to constantly wash their hands and using relaxation breathing to minimize or reduce their anxiety levels. Cognitive behavior techniques are also beneficial at helping the client

to rehearse the association between his thoughts, feelings, and behavioral responses.

PANDAS

PANDAS are Pediatric Autoimmune Neuropsychiatric Disorders associated with Group A Streptococci. The primary two disorders seen are OCD and Tic disorders (covered in Chapter 14). Murphy and Pichichero of the University of Rochester Medical Center identified 12 children with new onset PANDAS. They found that the mean age at presentation was 7, and there was a 4 to 1 ratio of males to females. All of these children developed a rapid onset of OCD or Tic disorder following a strep throat infection; parents could identify the exact day the symptoms began. Prior to this date, there was no evidence of any neuropsychiatric disorders in any of the children. In these children, 75% of the compulsions were germ-related, and more than half also had urinary urgency and frequency without infection. The children were treated with broad-spectrum antibiotics for 10 days, and the OCD symptoms resolved in 14 days. Six of the children relapsed and again had positive throat cultures for Group A strep. Recommendations of the study were that if a parent calls with reports of a sudden onset of strange behaviors in a child, and the child has had a recent sore throat or fever, than PANDAS should be considered and the child should be placed on a course of antibiotics. Currently it is not known if PANDAS is predictive of a later onset OCD or Tic disorder (Hughes, 2002).

NURSING MANAGEMENT OF THE ANXIOUS CLIENT

Clients with anxiety are commonly encountered in inpatient, outpatient, and general medical practice offices. Nurses can help by obtaining thorough histories that include symptoms and precipitating events. Anxiety disorders that can be tied to specific objects or events (e.g., PTSD, phobias, social anxiety) are sometimes easier to manage than are GAD and OCD. Pediatric nurses should be aware of PANDAS and ask parents about recent colds, fevers, or sore throats. Client education is beneficial as many clients with an anxiety disorder fear they are "going crazy." Providing reassurance that they have a relatively common medical condition may help to alleviate some of those fears. Talking with clients and their families about the "fight or flight" response will set the groundwork for relaxation and guided imagery training, and developing an exercise plan. Nurses can also advocate for the client with the prescribing practitioner. As tempting as is the immediate relief provided by benzodiazepines, they should be prescribed judiciously for the client. Most clients should be started on an SSRI or a TCA prescription (including children) and be provided limited benzodiazepines for p.r.n. usage only. In the primary care setting, clients with anxiety disorders need to be referred to counselors, particularly ones who specialize in cognitive behavior therapy techniques or have extra training in the treatment of PTSD. Nurses can help to facilitate these referrals and explain to the client and family the rationales for therapy. Hospitalized clients frequently have anxiety (in both the mental health and general medical population). Implementing relaxation techniques and providing p.r.n. medications will help. Establishing a rapport with the client is essential. Spending a little extra time actively listening to the client's concerns is as valuable for a client with anxiety as is catheter care to the postoperative client.

GENERALIZED ANXIETY DISORDER CASE STUDY

Casey is a 16-year-old girl who is being seen in the pediatrician's office for complaints of stomachaches nearly every day at school. She has been going to the nurse's office frequently and asking the health aid to call her mother. Occasionally she will also request an acetaminophen tablet for headaches. Casey was an honor roll student her freshman year, but this year her grades have dropped to a B-C average. During her appointment, she tells the nurse that she is worried that she won't be able to get into college with such poor grades. A college student was recently abducted while out riding her bicycle in Casey's hometown; she was later found murdered. Casey has been asking her mother to carry a cellular phone when she goes out jogging in the evenings, and she calls her every 15 minutes. When her mother doesn't return promptly in 45 minutes, Casey calls her cellular phone in a panic. One time she called 911 to report her mother as missing when the cellular phone batteries went dead. At home, Casey has reported trouble falling asleep at night before 1:00 a.m., and then she has vague nightmares of being chased by vampires and zombies from "The Night of the Living Dead." She feels tired during the day at school. Casey's parents divorced 14 years previously, but she has a stable home life at both her mother and her father's homes. Lately she hasn't wanted to go out with friends or leave home very often, unless her mother leaves with her (even then she really wants to remain at home). Medically, Casey is healthy. She has no allergies or history of any medical problems. She does not take any medications. She was a full-term infant and met all of her developmental milestones on target. There is a positive history of anxiety and depression on her mothers' side of the family, but none presently. The pediatrician diagnoses Casey with gastritis secondary to a generalized anxiety disorder. After consulting with the parents, she prescribes Zoloft® 50 mg once-daily plus Zantac® 150 mg at bedtime (h.s).

NURSING CARE PLAN

Problem Listing

- Stomachaches
- Headaches
- Nonspecific worries
- Social isolation
- Feelings of being unsafe
- Sleep disturbance
- Feelings that her family is unsafe

Priority Nursing Diagnosis

Anxiety related to perceived threats to integrity of self and family as evidenced by persistent worries, stomachaches, and a drop in academic performance.

Long-term Goal

Client will have anxiety reduced to a level that no longer interferes with her functioning.

Short-term Objectives

1. Client will report no stomachaches.
2. Client will stop calling mother every 15 minutes while jogging.
3. Client will bring grades back to the previous A-B average.

Nursing Interventions

1. Establish a sense of rapport and trust with the client by utilizing the active listening techniques of open-ended questions, clarifying, validating, and reflecting feelings.
2. Remain nonjudgmental and noncritical of the client.
3. Teach the client relaxation breathing to be utilized in times of stress. Practice these techniques until the client has mastered them.
4. Talk the client through a guided imagery session and teach how to utilize guided imagery when alone.
5. Consult with parents regarding client's need for reassurance and support.
6. Provide medication education for SSRIs.
7. Assist the client in developing a plan for completing homework in a timely manner.
8. Ask the client to keep a daily journal of thoughts and feelings, and how they impacted behavior for that day.
9. Encourage client to resume social activities with peers.

CHAPTER 10
Questions 64-70

64. *Eugene presents to the emergency department complaining of shortness of breath, trembling, feeling numb in his face and hands, and a sensation of choking. He thought he was having a heart attack.* The most likely cause of this client's symptoms is

   a. a dissociative episode.

   b. claustrophobia.

   c. a psychotic break.

   d. a panic attack.

65. Posttraumatic stress disorder symptoms may include

   a. problems being in a room full of people.

   b. repetitive and nonproductive behaviors.

   c. generalized fears of a variety of events or situations.

   d. hypervigilance and insomnia.

66. Repetitively checking to see that the windows are closed, the range is turned off, and the doors are locked is an example of

   a. generalized anxiety disorder.

   b. obsessive-compulsive disorder.

   c. posttraumatic stress disorder.

   d. panic disorder.

67. The type of therapy that involves reframing one's thoughts about events or situations in order to produce a more effective emotional and behavioral response is called

   a. cognitive behavior therapy.

   b. interpersonal therapy.

   c. psychoanalysis.

   d. behavioral modification.

68. Helping a client to imagine sitting on a beach, listening to the waves and feeling the warm sun is called

   a. cognitive behavior therapy.

   b. interpersonal therapy.

   c. behavior modification.

   d. guided imagery.

69. The usefulness of benzodiazepines is limited by

   a. their potential for habituation and dependency.

   b. a high risk of toxicity.

   c. the development of extrapyramidal syndrome symptoms.

   d. a lack of efficacy in anxiety disorders.

70. An SSRI that is specifically indicated for treating OCD is

   a. Tofranil®.

   b. Effexor XR®.

   c. Luvox®.

   d. Librium®.

CHAPTER 11

EATING, SLEEPING, AND SOMATOFORM DISORDERS

CHAPTER OBJECTIVE

At the end of this chapter, the reader will be able to recognize mental health disorders that are expressed by poor nutrition, medical complaints, or sleep problems.

LEARNING OBJECTIVES

By the completion of the chapter, the reader will be able to

1. describe symptoms of anorexia nervosa and bulimia.

2. differentiate somatoform disorders from other medical conditions.

3. recognize sleep disorders.

4. discuss relevant treatment for disorders involving health, nutrition, and sleep problems.

EATING DISORDERS

The *DSM-IV-TR* recognizes two types of eating disorders: anorexia nervosa and bulimia nervosa. Both are characterized by severe disturbances in eating behavior, often accompanied by body perception distortions. Eating disorders often begin in mid-late adolescence following a stressful life event. Severe cases may require hospitalization. Mortality related to anorexia nervosa is a little over 5% of diagnosed clients (the lifetime prevalence for anorexia nervosa is around 0.5%). Approximately 90% of all clients are female. Causes for an eating disorder are still unknown — but contributing factors include sociocultural pressures, family dynamics, and possibly biological issues. Images presented in the fashion or entertainment industry often portray the "ideal" body type as one with little to no fat. This sends a message to young women that they are "flawed" if they are unable to obtain this appearance. A character-type often seen in anorexia nervosa is a young woman with obsessive, perfectionistic tendencies, overly rigid or anxious coping responses, and enmeshed or controlling parents. There can be a familial component to the disorder as well with food and eating behaviors assuming an inappropriately over-important role in the family's interactions with one another.

Anorexia Nervosa

The essential feature of anorexia nervosa is a refusal to gain or maintain weight, accomplished primarily through starvation. Diagnostic criteria for anorexia nervosa include the following:

1. Refusal to maintain body weight at a minimally normal weight for age and height, or failure to make expected weight gains

2. Intense fear of gaining weight or becoming fat (even when underweight)

3. Disturbances in the way body shape or weight is experienced (i.e., undue influence on self-esteem, self-valuation, or denial of the seriousness of the problem)

4. Amenorrhea (in postmenarcheal clients), or the absence of at least three menstrual cycles

Subtypes of anorexia nervosa include restricting (absence of self-induced vomiting or misuse of laxatives, diuretics, or enemas) and binge eating/purging (presence of regular binge-eating or purging during an episode of anorexia).

Seriously underweight clients may manifest depression, irritability, insomnia, and social withdrawal. There may be concerns about eating in public, feelings of inadequacy, or an apparent lack of emotional expression. There is usually an obsession about food, which may take the form of hoarding. Clients with a binge eating/purging subtype are more likely to have a personality disorder (discussed in Chapter 12) or abuse substances. Other self-destructive behaviors may present, such as sexual promiscuity, self-mutilation, or suicide attempts. Relationships with family and peers can become strained and marked by conflict.

Physical findings associated with anorexia nervosa are attributable to starvation. In addition to amenorrhea, there are complaints of constipation, abdominal pain, cold intolerance, fatigue, and lethargy. Low blood pressure and body temperatures, and bradycardia may be found. Dry hair and skin, or hair loss are common. Some clients develop lanugo, which is a fine downy body hair similar to that seen in newborn infants. Peripheral edema, bruising or petechiae, enlarged parotid (salivary) glands, and a yellowing of the skin may occur. Clients who induce vomiting may have tooth enamel erosion or tooth loss. Later findings can include dehydration, osteoporosis, impaired renal function, cardiac arrhythmias, and congestive heart failure.

Bulimia Nervosa

In bulimia nervosa, binge eating and purging behaviors are seen, but without the severe dietary restrictions found in anorexia nervosa. The client's self-perception and evaluation are excessively influenced by body shape and weight.

A binge is defined as eating an excessive amount of food in a short period of time — usually less than 2 hours. Binge foods typically are high-calorie, sugary foods, such as ice cream or cake. Clients who binge are typically ashamed of the behavior and attempt to hide it. Binges are often precipitated by emotional stress, and are followed by feelings of self-criticism, guilt, and depression. A sense of lack of control usually accompanies the binging.

Purging occurs in response to feelings of shame and guilt. The most common form of purging is self-induced vomiting (80%-90%). The immediate gains from vomiting include relief from physical discomfort due to excessive intake, and a reduced fear of gaining weight. Other purging behaviors include the misuse of laxatives (30%), diuretics, or enemas. Excess exercising with the express purpose of "purging" calories is also a form of bulimia nervosa. Use of diet pills, diet aids, or even thyroid hormone supplements can also occur.

Medical complications due to binging may include significant and permanent tooth enamel loss, dental cavities, calluses or scars of the back of the hand, menstrual irregularities, bowel problems (with chronic laxative use), fluid and electrolyte imbalances, esophageal tears, gastric rupture, and cardiac arrhythmias. Low weight does not often occur — in fact, most clients with bulimia nervosa maintain their body weight.

NURSING MANAGEMENT OF THE CLIENT WITH AN EATING DISORDER

Nurses will usually encounter clients with anorexia nervosa in an inpatient setting. Clients with bulimia nervosa rarely require hospital care. Nurses need to work diligently to avoid seeming judgmental of the client. Active listening combined with consistent behavioral limitations helps to provide a sense of security and support. Staff should de-emphasize weighing the client more than necessary as this may promote control issues. Instead, the nurse should focus on feelings associated with eating (or binging/purging) and the associated consequences. Helping a client to develop awareness of the link between behavior and feelings may help to change the behavior in a positive manner. Calorie counts are usually necessary to determine actual food intake. The monitoring of electrolyte, calcium, and magnesium levels is important. Intravenous fluids or feeding tubes with liquid supplements may be needed for severe starvation. Observing for signs of purging is usually recommended. Encouraging light activity, and providing diet education helps to promote a healthy lifestyle. Support or therapy groups can be powerful tools as young adults/adolescents tend to be peer-oriented and the feedback from others is invaluable. Staff should expect the client to experience a good deal of anxiety with any weight gain — positive reinforcement for even small gains is extremely important.

Medication Interventions

There are no medications specifically indicated for the treatment of eating disorders. Commonly, vitamin and mineral supplementation is provided. Antidepressant medications are useful in helping to treat associated depression, mood swings, and anxiety symptoms. Anxiolytics may be used on an as needed (p.r.n.) basis.

ANOREXIA NERVOSA CASE STUDY

*B*rittany *is an attractive, petite cheerleader in the 8th grade. She wants to make the high school squad next year, but some of her friends tell her that the competition is really hard and you have to be perfect to get selected. Brittany goes through a*

growth spurt the summer before high school and she grows to 5'7" and puts on 10 lb, bringing her weight up to 135 lb. One of the boys from her school sees her at the mall, and says, "Hey, you been eating all summer or what?" Brittany becomes determined to lose weight. She starts to skip breakfast, then lunch. Soon she is eating once a day. She tells her family that she is going to be a vegetarian "because meat is gross." She starts exercising 2-3 hours every evening. Her weight starts to come off and she starts to get compliments from her friends. At 120 lb her mother suggests that she looks a little thin, but Brittany only sees fat around her thighs and stomach. Soon she is only eating a little lettuce (no dressing) and an apple for the day. Her weight continues to drop, and she notices some of her hair falling out in the shower. Although she is still exercising, she stops going out with friends because she is too tired. At 105 lb her menstrual cycles cease. By now, her parents are very concerned and they take her to a pediatrician. He tells them it's "just a phase, a lot of girls go through," so they try not to worry. By Christmas, Brittany weighs only 90 lb and she looks emaciated. She tells her best friend, Jennie, that she "just needs to lose a little more." At 84 lb Brittany faints at school and is rushed to the hospital. She is admitted to the intensive care unit for premature ventricular contractions and starvation syndrome. A psychiatric referral is made as well. Once stabilized, she is referred to an eating disorder specialist who meets with her and her family once a week to help Brittany develop some understanding of the disorder, and set a reasonable goal weight for maintenance.

NURSING CARE PLAN

Problem Listing

- Calorie intake less than body requirements
- Cardiac arrhythmia
- Amenorrhea

- Distorted body perception
- Low self-esteem

Priority Nursing Diagnosis

Alteration in nutrition, less than body requirements, related to self-induced eating disorder, as evidenced by a body weight of 84 lb with a height of 5'7".

Long-term Goal

Client will return to a body weight of 115 lb or above.

Short-term Objectives

1. Client will gain 1-2 pounds every week.
2. Client will eat a combination of carbohydrates, fats, and proteins.
3. Client will identify three positive qualities about self not related to physical appearance or weight.
4. Client will verbalize an understanding of the diet plan.

Nursing Interventions

1. Daily calorie count — instruct family and client for home usage.
2. Monitor fluid intake and electrolyte balances.
3. Educate the client about healthy food choices.
4. Provide support and encouragement with rewards for healthy weight gain.
5. Refer client to appropriate therapy (individual and group) and support services in the community.

SOMATOFORM DISORDERS

The common features of the somatoform disorders are the occurrence of physical symptoms in the absence of a diagnosed medical condition or substance abuse problem. The symptoms must cause clinically significant distress or functional impairment. Somatoform disorders are often encountered in general medical practices, and may account for numerous unnecessary tests, X-rays, hospitalizations, and even surgeries every year. Five types of somatoform disorders will be discussed here: somatization disorder, conversion disorder, pain disorder, hypochondriasis, and body dysmorphic disorder.

Somatization Disorder

A somatization disorder is one in which there is a pattern of recurring, multiple physical complaints that result in significant functional impairment, or medical intervention (including medications). Symptoms occur before age 30, and continue for years. Somatization disorders are seen more often in women, and they have a familial tendency. The men in these families tend to have a greater occurrence of substance dependence and antisocial personality disorder. Making the diagnosis of a somatization disorder requires ruling out all other medical causes, which may include disorders such as hypothyroidism, lupus erythematosus, arthritis, multiple sclerosis, or Lyme disease. *DSM-IV-TR* diagnostic criteria for somatization disorder include the following:

1. A history of many physical complaints over several years resulting in treatment being sought or significant functional impairment
2. Each of the following criteria must be met:
   a. four pain symptoms (e.g., headaches, joint pain, backaches)
   b. two gastrointestinal (GI) symptoms (e.g., nausea, gas, bloating, heartburn, vomiting, constipation, diarrhea)
   c. one sexual symptom (e.g., irregular menses, pain with intercourse, erectile dysfunction)
   d. one pseudoneurological symptom (e.g., impaired balance, weakness, trouble swallowing, numbness or tingling of extremi-

ties, double vision, blindness, fainting, paralysis)

3. Either (a) or (b)

   a. No medical cause found for the symptoms in criterion 2.

   b. In the presence of an actual medical condition, the symptoms or functioning of the client worsening more than what could be reasonably expected.

4. The symptoms not intentionally produced or feigned (as in factitious disorder or malingering)

An undifferentiated somatoform disorder may also occur where only one or two symptoms are present, and they persist for 6 months or longer. These symptoms include things such as chronic fatigue, loss of appetite, GI problems or urinary tract complaints.

Conversion Disorder

The essential features of a conversion disorder are the presence of symptoms that affect motor or sensory function, and that suggest a neurological disorder or other medical condition. To diagnose a conversion disorder, first rule out any legitimate medical conditions. Voluntary motor or sensory functions might include symptoms such as paralysis, blindness, deafness, seizures, weakness or falling, loss of touch or pain sensation, or impaired coordination. Conversion symptoms are often inconsistent and do not follow expected neurological pathways (e.g., a "paralyzed" arm will move during sleep). Electromyelograms and electroencephalograms (EEGs) will be normal. Psychologically, the conversion symptoms may be reflective of an underlying trauma or distress (e.g., the man who witnesses a murder may become "blind"). Although the client may receive secondary gains from the symptoms, in the form of increased attention and nurturance, it is important to note that these symptoms are not "faked" — that is, they are real to the client and quite distressful. Culturally

sanctioned symptoms, such as visions as a part of religious rituals are not considered to be conversion symptoms. Subtypes of conversion disorders include motor symptom or deficit (loss of voluntary muscle controls), sensory symptom or deficit (loss of touch, pain, eyesight, or hearing.), seizures or convulsions, and mixed presentation.

Pain Disorder

In a pain disorder, the pain must be the predominant focus of the client and it must cause clinically significant distress or interference with social, occupational, or other important areas of functioning. The pain is not intentionally produced or "faked" (as in factitious disorder and malingering), nor is it associated with psychosis, anxiety, or a depressive disorder. There may be accompanying medical conditions, but the pain must be the predominant concern and demonstrate chronicity in nature. Psychological factors have an important role in the onset, severity, exacerbation, or maintenance of the pain.

Hypochondriasis

A client with hypochondriasis is preoccupied with fears of having or developing a medical disorder. In many cases, personality traits exist where clients have a lifelong pattern of focusing on body symptoms and seeking medical advice. Clients with hypochondriasis may have intrusive thoughts and compulsive behaviors. Hypochondriasis differs from an obsessive-compulsive disorder (OCD), illness subtype in that with OCD, a client fears getting a disease whereas in hypochondriasis the client believes to have some, as yet undiagnosed, disease. *DSM-IV-TR* criteria include the following:

1. Preoccupation with a fear of having a serious disease based on bodily symptoms.

2. The preoccupation persists despite medical evaluation and reassurance.

3. The belief does not meet the criteria of being a delusion.

4. The belief causes clinically significant distress in various areas of functioning.

5. The duration is at least 6 months.

6. The preoccupation cannot be better accounted for by generalized anxiety disorder (GAD), OCD, panic disorder, major depression, or another psychiatric or substance abuse disorder.

Body Dysmorphic Disorder

A preoccupation with a defect in physical appearance is known as body dysmorphic disorder. The defect is either not present, or is so slight that the amount of preoccupation seen is extreme. There must be significant distress and impairment of functioning. Complaints seen may take the form of imagined flaws of the face or head (e.g., hair thinning, acne, wrinkles, vascular markings, swelling, or asymmetry) or other preoccupations such as the shape or size of body parts (e.g., eyes, ears, breasts, or penis). Any body part, or more than one, may be a focus. Because of severe embarrassment over the perceived flaw, clients may view themselves as ugly and feel unloveable. Thoughts about the "defect" may become significantly intrusive and negative, to the point that self-mutilation or suicide can occur. The client may try to hide the "defect" with clothing, beards, or hairstyles. Insight is often poor and some clients reach the point of becoming delusional. Clients with this disorder also often believe that everyone else is talking about the "defect" and feeling either disgust or pity for them. Clients may quit jobs or school, or stop going out of the house altogether. Clients with body dysmorphic disorder may go to extremes to try and alter the "defect" including steroid use with body building, plastic surgery, implants, or even self-surgery. Body dysmorphic disorder tends to be equally prevalent in men and women, and is higher in association with anxiety and depressive disorders. In cosmetic and dermatology settings, prevalence rates are as high as 6% to 15% (*DSM-IV-TR*).

NURSING MANAGEMENT OF THE CLIENT WITH A SOMATOFORM DISORDER

It is important for the nurse to realize that, unlike factitious disorders (where clients fabricate symptoms) or malingering (where clients lie about symptoms), clients with a somatoform disorder are in a great deal of distress. They truly believe that there is a medical problem and no one can, or will, help them. The best approach for the nurse is to provide support and compassion to the client. Frequently, health care providers are frustrated with clients that have no clear diagnosis and seem to be attention seeking, and they tend to shun them or disregard their complaints. A more helpful approach is to provide the client with nurturance and reassurance in order to forge a more collaborative relationship. Refocusing the client on strengths and abilities, rather than liabilities, will promote self-esteem. Assisting the client in identifying coping strategies will provide a sense of control for the client. Clients may be resistant to therapy, as they believe the problem to be medical and not psychological. The nurse can encourage the client to see a counselor in addition to any medical testing, on the rationale that the stress experienced by the medical symptoms certainly warrants additional support. A therapist can help the client identify the purpose that the symptoms serve, and to reframe or come up with other ways to get emotional needs of love and belonging met in the absence of an illness.

SOMATIZATION DISORDER CASE STUDY

Bertha is a 45-year-old divorced woman who has been going to physicians since she was 22 years old. Her ex-husband was abusive and an alcoholic. She suffers from chronic fatigue, headaches, diarrhea (or sometimes constipation), and funny tingling feelings in her legs, hot flashes, and dizziness. At age 25 she had a total abdominal hysterectomy for irregular cycles. Persistent abdominal pain resulted in an exploratory laparoscopy at age 27. Bertha also had a cholecystectomy and incidental appendectomy for small gallstones when she was age 32. When her surgical wound became infected and separated, she had to have a mesh placed. At home, she "takes to her bed" frequently with migraine headaches. Her three adolescent children are left to feed and care for themselves, with very little supervision. Bertha "threw out her back" carrying groceries one day last year, and she takes prescription pain medications several times a day. Most of her family won't visit anymore — they have grown tired of hearing her persistent complaining and tales of medical treatments gone awry. The rheumatologist put Bertha on nonsteroidal anti-inflammatory medications for her joint pain, the surgeon gave her antacids for her "heartburn," and her family doctor gives her hormone replacement plus sleeping pills (for her chronic insomnia). Bertha is increasingly depressed and doesn't understand why no one can tell her what is wrong with her. Her 16-year-old son came home from school to find her unconscious with empty pain pill bottles. She was rushed to the hospital and admitted to the intensive care unit.

NURSING CARE PLAN

Problem Listing

- Chronic pain — headaches, backaches, abdominal pain, joint pain
- GI symptoms — diarrhea, constipation, heartburn
- Sexual symptoms — hot flashes, surgically-induced menopause
- Neurological symptoms — weakness, numbness, and tingling extremities
- Psychological symptoms — depression, suicide attempt, low self-esteem

- Social problems — family rejection, no diversional activities, unemployed, children grown and more independent

Priority Nursing Diagnosis

Chronic low self-esteem related to long-standing reliance on others to meet her emotional needs as evidenced by the development of numerous physical ailments that require frequent medical evaluation.

Long-term Goal

Client will develop supportive relationships in the community to meet her needs for support and reassurance.

Short-term Objectives

1. Client will identify two activities that she can do on a weekly basis (may include volunteer work).
2. Client will be able to list at least three positive attributes.
3. Client will be able to have a 30-minute conversation with another adult and not discuss any physical complaints.
4. Client will report improved relationships with the three children.

Nursing Interventions

1. Assist the client in identifying community resources and volunteer opportunities.
2. Support the client in finding and listing three positive attributes.
3. Gently redirect the client away from physical complaints during conversations and toward social or life events.
4. Provide a nonjudgmental, caring approach.
5. Refer for family therapy for client and children.

SLEEP DISORDERS

Sleep disorders, or dyssomnias, are primary disorders of initiating or maintaining sleep, or of excessive sleepiness. The *DSM-IV-TR* recognizes several types: primary insomnia, primary hypersomnia, narcolepsy, breathing-related sleep disorder, and circadian rhythm sleep disorder. Each of these will be discussed individually along with recommended treatment. Dyssomnia disorder, not otherwise specified, is used for sleep disorders that do not fit into another, more specific category.

Primary Insomnia

Primary insomnia is a complaint of difficulty in initiating or maintaining sleep that lasts at least 1 month. There must be impairment in social, occupational, or other important areas of functioning as a result. The insomnia cannot be better accounted for by a substance abuse problem. Some clients claim to sleep, but feel that their sleep is not restful or restorative. Primary insomnia is often a combination of hyperarousal (due to physical, cognitive, or emotional concerns) and negative conditioning. The anxiety over chronic sleep problems may contribute to the development of a cycle where the anticipation of insomnia compounds the sleeping problem. Maladaptive sleep habits (e.g., daytime napping, following an erratic sleep schedule) can worsen the symptoms. Chronic insomnia may lead to fatigue, poor concentration, decreased attention to details, and moodiness (irritability or lability). "Short sleepers" are differentiated from insomnia in that the client requires less sleep to feel restful.

Nursing Management of Primary Insomnia

Combining medication intervention with sleep pattern restructuring is the most effective means of treating primary insomnia. Nursing interventions that may be useful are identified in Table 11-1 along with medications that are commonly utilized.

Primary Hypersomnia

Hypersomnia refers to excessive sleepiness for at least 1 month. Symptoms include either prolonged sleep or daytime sleep episodes occurring almost daily. The sleepiness must interfere with functioning in some manner, and it cannot be caused by another mental disorder or substance use. Clients with primary hypersomnia may sleep 8-12 hours, have difficulty waking up, and still feel sleepy during the day. Unintentional sleep episodes typically occur in low-stimulation situations, such as driving long distances, reading, attending lectures, or watching television. Episodes come on gradually rather than abruptly, and may be quite embarrassing for the client. Often, primary hypersomnia is associated with mild to moderate depression.

Narcolepsy

Narcolepsy involves repeated, irresistible attacks of refreshing sleep, cataplexy, and recurrent intrusions of rapid eye movement (REM) sleep into the transition period between sleep and wakefulness. The sleep attacks must occur daily over a period of at least 3 months. One or both of the following must also occur: Cataplexy (episodes of sudden, bilateral loss of muscle tone that last for seconds to minutes), or intrusive REM sleep with paralysis of voluntary muscles or dreamlike hallucinations. As with most other conditions, the presence of substance use or other medical or psychiatric condition must be ruled out. Narcolepsy episodes can be dramatic and occur in the middle of an activity or conversation. Episodes typically last 10-20 minutes, and may occur up to 6 times per day. Clients vary in their ability to "fight off" the sleep attacks. The symptom of cataplexy is often triggered by a strong emotion (laughter, anger, surprise) and may be mild (slight drooping of the eyelids) or dramatic (fall to the ground). Motor control is always regained. The symptoms of sleep paralysis (being aware of surroundings but

TABLE 11-1: NURSING INTERVENTIONS FOR PRIMARY INSOMNIA

1. Eliminate or significantly reduce caffeine (no more than two caffeine beverages daily, no caffeine after 5:00 p.m.).
2. Eliminate or significantly reduce alcohol intake (may interfere with REM sleep stages).
3. Set the alarm clock and get up at the same time every day.
4. Eliminate daytime napping.
5. Perform light exercises daily — but not within 2 hours of bedtime.
6. Have a light snack in the evening — avoid heavy foods within 2 hours of bedtime.
7. Sleep with the lights off and curtains or shades drawn.
8. Keep the room temperature comfortably warm in the winter, cool in the summer.
9. Consider use of "white noise" (electric fan, water fountain, sound machine).
10. Avoid television or "talk" radio.
11 Go to bed at the same time. Read or listen to acoustic music. If not asleep in 20 minutes, try as needed (p.r.n.) medications (see below).
12. Do not use the bedroom for working, studying, or performing other mentally challenging activities.

MEDICATION INTERVENTIONS

Category	Generic Name	Trade Name	Comments
Antihistamine	Diphenhydramine	Benadryl®, Tylenol PM®	Safe, gentle agent. Drowsiness is a side effect.
Alternative	Melatonin	Melatonex®	Hormone produced in response to sunlight. Bizarre dreams can occur.
Benzodiazepine	Temazepam	Restoril®	Potential for dependency
	Flurazepam	Dalmane®	Potential for dependency
	Triazolam	Halcion®	Potential for dependency, psychosis
Nonbenzodiazepine	Zaleplon	Sonata®	Potential for habituation
	Zolpidem	Ambien®	Potential for habituation
Miscellaneous	Trazodone Chloral hydrate	Desyrel® Noctec®	Mild antidepressant. Extremely sedating. Good for 1-2 nights only.

unable to move) and hallucinatory dreams are thought to be due to REM sleep intrusions.

Research into narcolepsy and cataplexy at the Stanford Medical School Center for Narcolepsy, has identified some significant genetic markers for the disorder (www-med.stanford.edu). Additionally, sleep studies have identified a correlation between REM sleep abnormalities and the occurrence of the disorder.

Treatment for narcolepsy and cataplexy involves medications. Stimulant-type medications are indicated for the "sleep attacks." These include the following:

- Methylphenidate (Ritalin®, Ritalin SR®, Methadate CD®, Concerta®)
- Dexamphetamine (Dexedrine®, Dextrostat®)
- Dexamphetamine-salts (Adderall®, Adderall XR®)
- Methamphetamine HCl (Desoxyn®)
- Pemoline (Cylert®)
- Modafinil (Provigil®)

Side effects to stimulant medications include insomnia, jitteriness, tachycardia, decreased appetite, and irritability. The symptoms of abnormal REM sleep (cataplexy, sleep-wake hallucinations, sleep paralysis) are better treated with antidepressant medications

- Fluoxetine (Prozac®)
- Venlafaxine (Effexor®, Effexor XR®)
- Protriptyline (Vivactil®)
- Imipramine (Tofranil®)
- Desipramine (Norpramin®)
- Clomipramine (Anafranil®)

Side effects to these medications are specific to the category selective serotonin reuptake inhibitors (SSRIs), tricyclic antidepressants (TCAs). A thorough discussion of antidepressants appears in Chapter 8.

Breathing-related Sleep Disorder

Breathing-related sleep disorders, also known as "sleep apnea" are problems in sleep associated with abnormalities of ventilation and respiration. The most common presenting complaint among individuals is excess daytime sleepiness. Sleepiness results from frequent wakening during the night as the client attempts to breathe normally. Breathing-related sleep disorder consists of three subtypes: obstructive sleep apnea (usually seen in overweight individuals, also in children with enlarged adenoids and tonsils), central sleep apnea (cessation of breathing during sleep without obstruction), and central alveolar hypoventilation syndrome (waking occurs due to low oxygenation usually secondary to morbid obesity). Clients may complain of chest pain, choking, suffocation feelings, or anxiety. Clients with obstructive problems typically snore extremely loud. They may have difficulty awakening and report headaches. Dry mouth and thirst will lead to nocturia — compounding the problem. The daytime sleepiness can lead to mood changes, poor concentration, memory problems, irritability, and personality changes. Children with a breathing-related sleep disorder may present as extremely hyperactive or aggressive, with poor attention span and concentration — leading to an initial diagnosis of attention-deficit/hyperactivity disorder.

Treatment for breathing-related sleep disorders involves identifying the cause through sleep-studies utilizing EEG readings. Surgery to remove tonsils and adenoids may be recommended. Weight loss will reduce both obstructive and hypoventilation types. Often, a continuous positive airway pressure (CPAP) machine is prescribed. The CPAP is a device that consists of an airway mask worn by the client during sleep, which provides either room air or a mixture of air plus oxygen in a small, continuously pressurized system. This serves to "hyperoxygenate" the alveoli of the lungs to keep blood (thus brain) levels of oxygen within a normal range.

Circadian Rhythm Sleep Disorder

Formerly referred to as a sleep-wake schedule disorder, circadian rhythm disorder is a persistent or recurrent pattern of sleep disturbance relative to a discrepancy between a client's sleep-wake urges and the ability to follow those patterns based on societal expectations. Four subtypes exist: delayed sleep phase (normal sleep at socially unacceptable hours, e.g., 4:00 a.m.-12:00 p.m.), jet lag (sleep requirements for a new time zone), shift work (adjusting to a night-shift schedule or a variable shift schedule), and unspecified (any others including an advanced sleep phase where the individual falls asleep early then wakens early, e.g., 6:00 p.m.-2:00 a.m.). Familial patterns have been identified for both delayed sleep and advanced sleep subtypes. Treatment consists of following sleep hygiene recommendations (Table 11-1) and utilizing sleep aids at the designated hour of sleep. Jet lag is frequently treated with melatonin supplements. Melatonin is a hormone secreted normally by the body in response to daylight hours, and it may be associated with seasonal affective disorder.

EXAM QUESTIONS

CHAPTER 11
Questions 71-77

71. Diagnostic criteria for anorexia nervosa include

    a. self-induced vomiting.

    b. disturbances in the way body shape or weight is experienced.

    c. a dysfunctional family system.

    d. a weight loss of 20% or the total basal metabolic index (BMI).

72. Bulimia is characterized by

    a. restricting intake to the point of starvation.

    b. gagging oneself to induce vomiting.

    c. self-mutilating behaviors.

    d. eating an excessive amount of food, then trying to purge it.

73. Diagnostic criteria for somatization disorder include

    a. two pain symptoms and several psycho-neurological symptoms.

    b. at least four GI symptoms accompanied by pain.

    c. a sexual abuse history accompanied by seizures.

    d. four pain symptoms, two GI symptoms, one sexual symptom, and one psycho-neurological symptom.

74. A client with hypochondriasis has

    a. an obsession with cleanliness and germ prevention.

    b. an irrational belief that they have an undiagnosed disease.

    c. a belief that a body part is defective.

    d. numerous drug-seeking behaviors.

75. A difficulty in initiating or maintaining sleep that lasts at least 1 month is known as

    a. hypersomnia.

    b. primary insomnia.

    c. narcolepsy.

    d. sleep-cycle disturbance.

76. The best nursing approach for the client with a somatoform disorder is to

    a. be confrontive and set firm limits.

    b. be supportive and compassionate.

    c. avoid becoming overly attached.

    d. maintain a technological focus.

77. An important nursing intervention for primary insomnia would be to

    a. set the alarm clock for the same time every day.

    b. encourage liberal use of at bedtime (h.s.) sedatives.

    c. tell the client to stay in bed "as long as it takes."

    d. advise the client to stop working night shifts.

CHAPTER 12

DOMESTIC VIOLENCE, DISSOCIATION, AND PERSONALITY DISORDERS

CHAPTER OBJECTIVE

At the end of this chapter, the reader will be able to discuss problems associated with domestic violence and how they relate to the development of dissociative and personality disorders.

LEARNING OBJECTIVES

Upon completing this chapter, the reader will be able to

1. describe the power and control wheel and how it relates to domestic violence.

2. recognize signs of childhood sexual abuse.

3. differentiate and describe the dissociative disorders.

4. recognize the various expressions of a personality disorder.

5. discuss nursing management for clients who have personality disorders.

VIOLENCE AND TRAUMA

Violence permeates our society. Assaults, rapes, and murders increase annually proportionate to population growth with rates highest in poorer, urban areas. Workplace violence is of particular concern to nursing with up to 48% of all nonfatal assaults taking place in health care facilities (National Institute for Occupational Safety and Health, 1997). Rape and sexual assault occur highest to women between the ages of 16 and 19, but underreporting may be as high as 30%. Ritual abuse, torture, or cult-related mind control are still present and usually affect children or young men and women. Perhaps the most devastating abuse of all does not occur in response to terrorism or outside forces, but is within the home itself. A family history of violence, abuse (physical or emotional), neglect, or sexual molestation can emotionally and psychologically cripple a person leading to years of dysfunctional relationships, acting-out behaviors, substance dependence, and depression. For the purposes of this book, two forms of violence will be discussed: domestic partner abuse and childhood sexual abuse.

DOMESTIC PARTNER ABUSE

Most portrayals of domestic partner abuse involves the male as perpetrator. In more than 90% of the time, this is the case (although the remaining 10% should be kept in mind). Partner-abuse victims tend to conceal their situation. Fear, shame and guilt play a major role in perpetuating the abuse. Some women who are abused do not feel they can support themselves and their children; however, a vast number of clients are intelligent or well educated and still can find themselves in an abusive relationship. To understand how this can

FIGURE 12-1: THE POWER AND CONTROL WHEEL

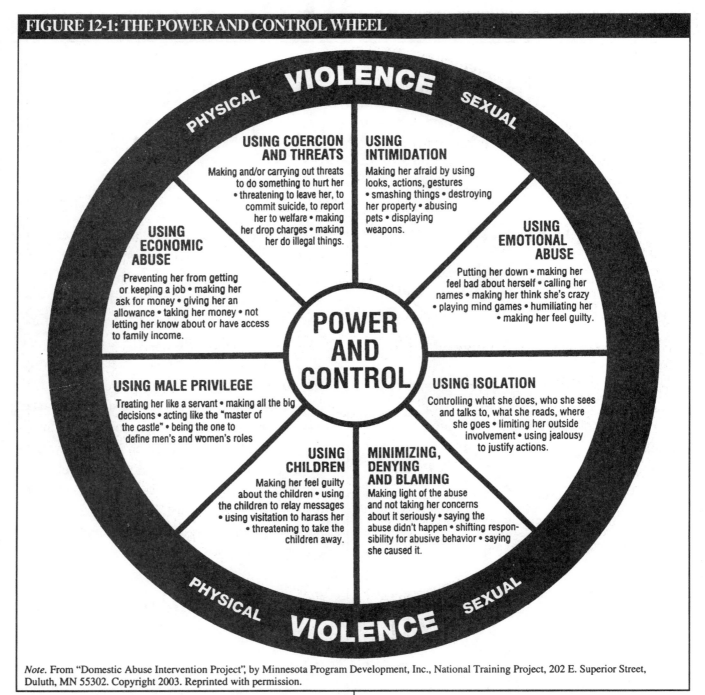

Note. From "Domestic Abuse Intervention Project", by Minnesota Program Development, Inc., National Training Project, 202 E. Superior Street, Duluth, MN 55302. Copyright 2003. Reprinted with permission.

occur, as well as why a woman would remain in an abusive relationship, it is helpful to look at the Power and Control Wheel developed by the Domestic Abuse Intervention Project in Duluth, Minnesota.

Before any physical violence occurs, numerous small steps will "condition" the couple and lead them toward a path of abuse. The Power and Control Wheel (Figure 12-1) divides abuse into parts, each of which has increasingly oppressive

and controlling behaviors leading eventually to physical or sexual assault.

A partner to the Power and Control Wheel is the Equality Wheel (Figure 12-2). The Equality Wheel addresses each of the areas of intimidation, threats, and abuse outlined in the Power and Control Wheel, but presents the clients with healthier options: "Using emotional abuse" is supplanted with "Respect," "Minimizing, denying, and blaming" is replaced by "Honesty and Accountability,"

FIGURE 12-2: THE EQUALITY WHEEL

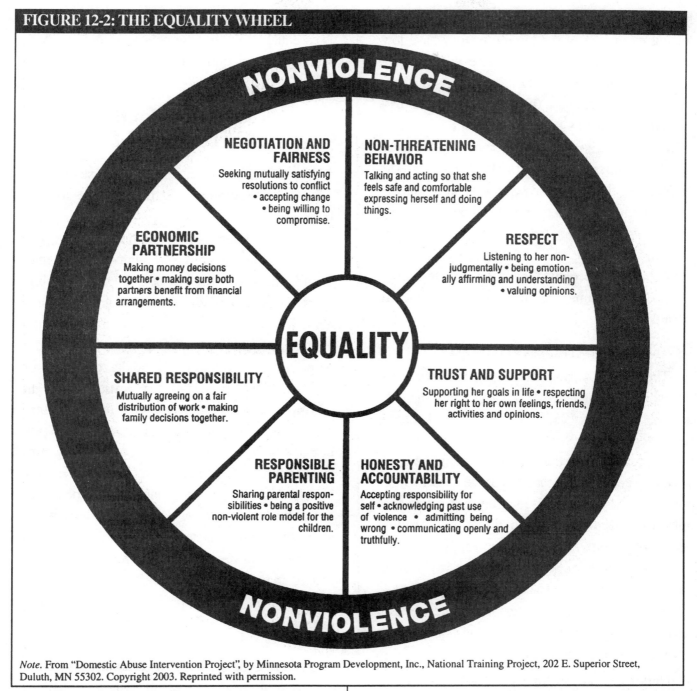

Note. From "Domestic Abuse Intervention Project", by Minnesota Program Development, Inc., National Training Project, 202 E. Superior Street, Duluth, MN 55302. Copyright 2003. Reprinted with permission.

and "Negotiation and Fairness" are taught as alternatives to "Using coercion and threats."

The effects on the client of being in a domestic abuse situation are to produce a learned hopelessness and helplessness, resignation and "giving up" feeling. Fear of death is warranted as 30-50% of women murdered in the United States are killed when they attempt to leave a domestic violence situation (3% of all male homicides are committed by abused partners in self-defense) (Keltner, Schwecke, & Bostrom, 2003). During the early stages of abuse, the male partner is often extremely apologetic and genuinely remorseful. He may promise "it will never happen again" and purchase gifts to bring them back together. After this honeymoon phase, the violence tends to escalate both in frequency and intensity. Women stay in abusive relationships for a variety of reasons: they feel at fault; they still love their partner; they were raised to be submissive; they have no family willing to help; they are afraid of being alone; they are protecting the image of the family; or they have low self-esteem. Stopping this cycle will usually require legal intervention. Long-term consequences of chronic partner abuse (if survived) lead to a phenomenon known as battered woman's syndrome, which is similar to the posttraumatic stress disorder (PTSD) discussed in Chapter 10. Victims report nightmares, flashbacks, hyperarousal states, recurrent fear, chronic anxiety, emotional detachment or numbness, insomnia, guilty feelings, low self-esteem, depression, and difficulty concentrating. It is important to recognize that the symptoms are a result of the trauma, and to work with the victim toward recovery.

Domestic Violence Interventions

The Duluth Abuse Intervention Project recognizes domestic violence as a societal, not individual, problem. Intervention is geared toward changing the community's response to violence by providing protection for the victim and using the legal system to change the behaviors of the abuser. Once perpetrators are convicted, they are given the option of attending psychoeducational groups instead of prison to develop better insight into their behaviors and learn new tools to cope with life. Failing to complete the classes will result in a revocation of probation and incarceration. Safety of the victim is always foremost and child visitations may be restricted (or supervised).

Nurses can provide valuable assistance as well. Abused women and their partners are frequently encountered in emergency department settings or community office settings. It is important to remain nonjudgmental and supportive while performing physical assessments to determine the extent of the abuse. Safety is of utmost importance — unlike with children or elderly clients, there is no governmental institution for reporting domestic abuse. Letting the victim know the options for shelter and treatment by providing phone numbers and

addresses for crisis centers or emergency housing is essential. Notifying the police can only be done with the consent of the victim.

CHILDHOOD SEXUAL ABUSE

The number of clients sexually abused as children is not known. Estimates have gone as high as 20% for girls and 7% for boys in some reports. It is likely that males underreport abuse due to embarrassment and shame. Abuse may include incest (relatives as perpetrators), fondling, intercourse, voyeurism, or exhibitionism. Victims come from every economic and social background, cultural and ethnic group. Childhood sexual abuse perpetrators are often trusted adults, teenagers, or older children. The relationship is usually thought of (initially) as supportive, trusting, or loving. There is always an imbalance in power — the perpetrator is able to persuade or coerce the victim through threats, intimidation, or fear. Children may be told that their parents or siblings will be killed, or that they will be "taken away" if they tell anyone about the abuse. Substance use contributes to the occurrence of sexual abuse. The child who is abused may have serious conflicting feelings — there may be physical pain, fear, and confusion intermingled with a feeling of being "special" or "the favorite." Behaviors that may indicate a child or an adolescent is being abused are listed in Table 12-1. Children who grow up with sexual abuse often have difficulty in discriminating emotional love from control and sex, and may end up with abusive partners as adults. Trust issues are significant in the adult client who has survived childhood abuse. PTSD (covered in Chapter 11) is frequently seen in adult survivors. Symptoms of PTSD are what will commonly lead the client to therapy. There has usually been a history of avoidance, unstable relationships, emotional numbing, or self-destructive behaviors (including substance depen-

TABLE 12-1: BEHAVIORS INDICATIVE OF CHILDHOOD SEXUAL ABUSE

Child	Adolescent
Sleep disturbances	Acting-out
Nightmares	Truancy
Refusal to sleep in own bed	Runaway
Eating disorders	Sexual promiscuity
Enuresis	Violent behaviors
Blood-stained underwear	Anger and rage
Recurrent urinary tract infections	Depression guilt
Vaginal yeast infections	Anxiety
Refusal to bathe	Substance abuse
Bedwetting	Prostitution
Encopresis	Early pregnancy
Anxiety symptoms	Early marriage
Anger	Perpetrating against others
Irritability	Self-mutilation
Depressive symptoms	Suicidal behaviors
Aggression in play	Regression
Sexualized play activities	Depersonalization
Masturbation	Dissociation
Poor impulse control	Impaired relationships
Self-destructive behaviors	
Perpetrating against younger children	

dence) prior to presentation. Repression can occur. Repression is a selective amnesia where events that become too overwhelming for the client to deal with are buried in the subconscious and "forgotten." Repression is not the same as suppression — where memories are painful but easily retrieved. In true repression, the client will not have any recollection of the events, and attempting to recover those traumatic memories can result in anxiety, panic attacks, or dissociation, which is a mental separation from reality similar to psychosis.

During dissociative episodes, clients may not know where they are, and may attempt to reenact abusive situations. Fear and panic are intense. The client can become agitated and violent toward others requiring emergency intervention. Dissociative disorders will be discussed in more depth in the following section.

Nursing management of the sexually-abused child or adolescent will be geared toward the symptoms and needs of the client. Support and maintaining safety is foremost. The health care provider must report any suspicions of abuse (sexual or physical) by calling the appropriate agencies, usually the Child Protective Service (CPS) division of the Office of Family and Children. Reporting abuse is a federal law. Choosing not to report can result in legal action and loss of any professional licenses. Child Protective Services will take the information (which should include name of victim, suspected circumstances, address where the victim can be found, and relevant phone numbers) and immediately send an investigator to interview the child. If the case is found to be substantiated (meaning there is significant evidence), then the child and siblings will be taken into custody and placed in foster care. Child Protective Services will obtain emergency CHINS status (Child in Need of Services) that makes the legal guardian of the child the county agency. The suspected perpetrator may be arrested. The non-perpetrating parent can also be arrested for "failure to protect" if there is evidence that the parent had knowledge of the abuse and did nothing to prevent it. Other interventions might include allowing the child to stay at home but ordering the suspected adult to leave while an investigation is underway, or allowing the child to stay with grandparents or other relatives. If the case is unsubstantiated, Child Protective Services will file it with no other action. Adolescents may present a difficult situation. Age 16 is considered to be the "age of consent" for adolescents to engage in sexual activity. Child Protective Services will rarely intervene once a child reaches this age unless other factors are present, such as a mental handicap of the child, a vast discrepancy in age between child and perpetrator (e.g., a 16-year-old girl having relations with a 30-year-old man), or if the alleged perpetrator is a family member.

Nursing care of the adult client who has been sexually abused combines providing empathy and support with setting limits on self-injurious behaviors. Directly asking about abuse during a nursing assessment is important, as the client may not be forthcoming. Examples of questions the nurse may ask could include "Were you ever molested as a child?" or "What's the worst thing that's ever happened to you in your life?" Assessing for memory lapses will help to determine if repression and dissociation are present. Teaching relaxation and stress management techniques to use during anxiety or panic attacks will be helpful. Making referrals to appropriate therapists or support groups (that specialize in sexual abuse trauma) will be necessary. Medications are usually indicated based on the symptoms presented. Anxiolytics may be needed for the anxiety and panic, antidepressants may be needed for depression, and antipsychotics for dissociation. Monitoring for substance abuse or dependence and providing safe detoxification services are appropriate, when indicated.

DISSOCIATIVE DISORDERS

The primary feature of a dissociative disorder is a disruption in the functions of consciousness, memory, identity, or perception. Dissociative disorders can onset rapidly, or more insidiously. They may persist for a short time or on a chronic basis. The *DSM-IV-TR* recognizes five dissociative disorders, which include dissociative disorder, not otherwise specified. The following four will be discussed: dissociative amnesia, dissociative fugue, dissociative identity disorder (formerly known as multiple personality disorder), and depersonalization disorder.

Dissociative Amnesia

The predominant concern of dissociative amnesia is an inability to recall important personal information. The memories lost are usually of a traumatic or highly stressful situation. The extent of memory loss is too great to be explained by forgetfulness. Localized amnesia refers to an inability to recall events in a specific time period — as with an automobile accident. In selective amnesia, generalities are remembered, but specifics may not be (e.g., violent combat experiences). Localized and selective amnesia are relatively common. Less common (but sensationalized on television and in movies) are generalized, continuous, and systematized amnesia. In generalized amnesia, clients cannot remember any of their life's events and may present for emergency care in a frightened state. Continuous amnesia refers to an inability to recall events from a specific time up to the present. It is ongoing — a client may not remember what occurred the day before. Finally, in systematized amnesia certain groups or characteristics (such as family members) cannot be remembered. Clients experiencing an amnesia disorder frequently experience depression, anxiety, depersonalization, trance-like states, and age regression. Impaired social relationships occur. The client may be more suggestible to hypnosis in therapy settings than individuals with other diagnoses.

Dissociative Fugue

A dissociative fugue state is characterized by sudden, unexpected travel away from one's home or customary activities, accompanied by an inability to remember some or all of one's past. There is usually confusion regarding identity, and the client may assume a new identity. The period of travel may be only hours, or as long as months. During a fugue, the client does not appear to be suffering from any clinical abnormalities such as depression or psychosis. Although rare, if a new identity is assumed it is usually a more outgoing and uninhibited type than the baseline personality. After the fugue state ends, traumatic events may be recalled (or selective amnesia may be present) and the client can experience depression, anxiety, grief, guilt, shame, and other forms of psychological distress. Certain cultural groups have "running" syndromes seen as a sudden onset of a high level of activity, a trancelike state, potentially dangerous running behaviors, and ultimate exhaustion, sleep and amnesia (Appendix A).

Dissociative Identity Disorder

Perhaps one of the most popularized, and most rare, forms of psychiatric disturbance is the dissociative identity disorder, formerly known as multiple personality disorder. In a dissociative identity disorder, two or more distinct identities or personality states are present that recurrently take control of a client's behavior. Important personal information may be forgotten. In children, the symptoms cannot be attributed to imaginary playmates or other fantasy play. Each personality state may be experienced as if it has a separate personal history, self-image, and even age. Often, the individual personalities assume different aspects of a "whole" person (i.e., one is aggressive, one is playful and impulsive, one is studious and responsible, one is promiscuous), and will emerge at times when their particular "talents" are needed. The client with this disorder will experience frequent memory gaps of personal history. Usually, the client will not have knowledge or awareness of the other personality states — although the other personalities may "know" each other. Transitions or "switching" usually occur at times of psychological stress. Behavioral manifestations will include rapid blinking, facial changes, disrupted thoughts, mannerism changes, or voice changes. Fifty percent of reported cases have 10 or fewer personality states;

although up to 100 have been documented (*DSM-IV-TR*).

Clients with dissociative identity disorder frequently report a history of severe physical, emotional, and sexual abuse starting early in childhood. Clients may demonstrate a number of PTSD symptoms (nightmares, flashbacks, depression, or hypervigilance), suicidal or self-mutilation behaviors, or aggression. Relationships with others are often dysfunctional. Eating disorders, sexual disorders, and other problems may be present. Clients with this disorder report migraine headaches and other stress-related physical problems. Different personality states may also have different physical responses such as pain tolerance or even conversion disorders (e.g., blindness).

Depersonalization Disorder

A depersonalization disorder is a persistent or recurrent experience of feeling detached from (or observing) one's own body or mental processes. The client may report feeling as if in a dream state. During the depersonalization experience, reality orientation remains intact and the client can respond to others. Age of onset is around 16, and clients usually report another more distressful symptom such as panic attacks or depression. Depersonalization symptoms are usually precipitated by severe stress, and they develop in nearly one-third of clients exposed to life-threatening danger (e.g., auto accidents, military combat, victim of a crime). Client may report a sensation of being out of control of their body or thoughts. A lack of emotional response and sensory anesthesia can occur (feeling numb all over). Depersonalization experiences are common, and a diagnosis should only be made if the symptoms cause a marked impairment in functioning.

TREATMENT OF DISSOCIATIVE DISORDERS

Therapy will usually take years and may involve some form of hypnosis by a trained hypnotherapist. Establishing trust between caregiver and client is essential. Ultimately, the client's mental state is extremely fragile during a dissociative disorder. Recovering memories can be painful, especially if the forgotten events were particularly traumatic. Providing a secure, safe environment during these episodes will be necessary to prevent the client from potentially harming the self or others. The goal in dissociative identity disorders is eventual reintegration of the client. Clinician opinions vary on how to address or converse with the other personality states — in general the nurse should not promote further splitting of the client by encouraging communication with altered states. Medications are not specifically indicated for dissociative disorders; however, clients may be treated for concomitant anxiety, panic attacks, or depression. Antipsychotics are sometimes prescribed.

PERSONALITY DISORDERS

Personality disorders are classified by the *DSM-IV-TR* as "Axis II" disorders. This means that they are not usually the primary focus of treatment, rather they are traits or characteristics of the client that tend to be dysfunctional and counterproductive for fitting into society. Personality disorders tend to be culture-specific. A client with a personality disorder may or may not feel that something is "wrong"; in fact, often the client believes that the problems in social relationships lie in other people. General diagnostic criteria for a personality disorder include the following:

1. A pattern of behavior that deviates markedly from the expectations of the client's culture manifested in two or more of the following areas:

   a. cognition — ways of perceiving and interpreting self, other people, and events

   b. affectivity — range, intensity, lability, and appropriateness of emotional responses

   c. interpersonal functioning

   d. impulse control

2. The pattern is inflexible and pervasive across a broad range of situations

3. The pattern leads to clinically significant distress

4. The pattern is stable and of long duration (at least to adolescence or early adulthood)

5. The pattern cannot be accounted for by another mental disorder (e.g., paranoid symptoms in schizophrenia)

6. The pattern cannot be due to the direct effects of alcohol or drugs

Causes for personality disorders were traditionally thought to be based in childhood experiences and learned behaviors in the family. Newer biological theories, based on twin studies and longitudinal family studies, suggest that some personality traits may be inherited (Keltner et al., 2003). The *DSM-IV-TR* recognizes 10 distinct personality disorders, with an 11th diagnosis of personality disorder, not otherwise specified. Personality disorders are further divided into subtypes or "clusters" as demonstrated in Table 12-2. An overview of these disorders follows.

Paranoid Personality Disorder

A paranoid personality disorder is seen in a client who demonstrates a pattern of pervasive distrust and suspiciousness of others. Paranoia due to alcohol, drugs, or a major disturbance, such as schizophrenia or dementia, must be ruled out. Four or more of the following symptoms must be present:

1. suspects (without basis) that others are exploiting or deceiving him

2. has unjustified doubts about the loyalty or trustworthiness of friends/family

3. is reluctant to confide in others for fear the information will be used against him

4. reads hidden messages into benign remarks or events

5. persistently bears grudges

6. perceives character or reputation attacks, and is quick to anger or retaliate

7. has recurrent, unjustified suspicions regarding fidelity of spouse or partner

Clients with paranoid personalities can be unpleasant if not frightening to live with. Always vigilant to insults and quick to react, this type of person can become agitated and violent with little provocation.

TABLE 12-2: SUBTYPE CLUSTERS OF PERSONALITY DISORDERS

Cluster A
Characterized by distinctly odd or eccentric behaviors
　1. Paranoid
　2. Schizoid
　3. Schizotypal

Cluster B
Characterized by overly dramatic, emotional or erratic behaviors
　1. Antisocial
　2. Borderline
　3. Histrionic
　4. Narcissistic

Cluster C
Characterized by chronically anxious or fearful behaviors
　1. Avoidant
　2. Dependent
　3. Obsessive-compulsive

Schizoid Personality Disorder

Individuals with schizoid personality disorders often seem indifferent to the approval or opinions of others, and they have a detachment from social relationships. These clients seem to lack a desire for intimacy or relationships with others. They are not bothered by insults or criticism, or buoyed up by praise or rewards. The person with a schizoid personality may demonstrate a limited range of emotional expression and affect. To make this diagnosis, at least four of the following must be seen:

1. neither desires nor enjoys close relationships (including family)

2. chooses solitary activities

3. has little interest in sexual activities with another person

4. takes pleasure in very few activities

5. lacks close friends or confidants

6. appears indifferent to praise or criticism

7. shows emotional coldness, flattening, or detachment

Goals may be vague and schizoid clients may seem to "drift" through life with little aim or direction.

Schizotypal Personality Disorder

In contrast to a schizoid personality disorder, the client with a schizotypal personality disorder demonstrates a pervasive pattern of social and interpersonal deficits marked by discomfort and a reduced capacity for relationships, accompanied by cognitive distortions or behavior eccentricities. Superstitions, unusual beliefs, or preoccupation with paranormal experiences may be seen. Thoughts may contain a magical component. Dress or mannerisms may be described as "odd." Diagnostic criteria require at least five of the following:

1. ideas of reference (not delusions)

2. odd beliefs or magical thinking that influences behavior

3. unusual perceptual experiences

4. odd thinking and speech

5. suspiciousness or paranoid ideation

6. inappropriate affect

7. behavior or appearance that is odd or eccentric

8. lack of close friends or confidants

9. excessive social anxiety (associated with paranoid fears)

Clients diagnosed with a schizotypal personality disorder occasionally will progress to developing more traditional symptoms indicative of schizophrenia.

Antisocial Personality Disorder

Also known as a sociopath, an individual with an antisocial personality disorder lacks the ability to have empathy for others, and persistently violates the rights of others. The disorder may begin in childhood when it is diagnosed as a "conduct disorder." Clients with antisocial personality are often charismatic criminals who may feel special entitlements are owed them by society. Diagnostic criteria for an antisocial personality disorder must include at least three of the following elements, and must occur by age 15 (but cannot be diagnosed prior to age 18):

1. failure to conform to social norms with respect to obeying the law

2. deceitfulness (lying, using aliases, conning others for profit)

3. impulsivity or failing to plan ahead

4. irritability and aggressiveness (repeated physical fights or assaults)

5. reckless disregard for the safety of others or self

6. irresponsibility in work behaviors, or financial obligations

7. lack of remorse or rationalizing that others "deserve it"

Clients with antisocial personalities are frequently seen in the prison system. Currently there are no good psychological treatments to change these character traits and the protection of society may be warranted.

Borderline Personality Disorder

Clients with borderline personality disorders demonstrate a pervasive pattern of unstable and erratic relationships. They tend to view the world in terms of "black or white," and they make dramatic efforts to avoid perceived abandonment by others. Gender-identity and other identity issues may be present. Both emotions and behaviors may be extremely labile and unpredictable. Suicide gestures, self-mutilation, and substance abuse problems are frequent. To make a diagnosis of borderline personality disorder, at least five of the following criteria must be met:

1. frantic efforts to avoid real or imagined abandonment

2. a pattern of unstable and intense interpersonal relationships demonstrating extremes of idealization and devaluation

3. unstable self-image or sense of self (identity disturbance)

4. impulsivity in at least two areas that are self-destructive (e.g., reckless driving, dangerous sexual practices, eating disorders)

5. suicidal behaviors, gestures or threats, or self-mutilating behaviors

6. marked mood instability

7. chronic feelings of emptiness

8. inappropriate or uncontrollable anger

9. transient, stress-induced paranoia, or dissociative episodes

Borderline personality disordered clients can be the most difficult of all psychiatric clients. They will go to great lengths to engineer discord among staff members, and attempt to "split" staff into disagreements over aspects of treatment planning such as therapy needs, discharge planning, and milieu management.

Histrionic Personality Disorder

Attention-seeking behaviors and excessive emotionality are the hallmarks of a histrionic personality disorder. Clients with this personality type tend towards manipulation of others and crave excitement or stimulation. They may enact a role of victim in interpersonal relationships. At least five of the following *DSM-IV-TR* criteria must be met to diagnose a histrionic personality disorder:

1. discomfort in situations where they are not the center of attention

2. interactions are often characterized by seductive or provocative behaviors

3. displays rapidly shifting and shallow emotions

4. uses physical appearance to draw attention to self

5. speech is excessively impressionistic and lacking in detail

6. exaggerated emotions, or theatrical or dramatized emotions

7. easily influenced by others or circumstances (suggestible)

8. considers relationships more intimate than they really are

Although emotional reactivity is seen, clients with histrionic personalities will often lack the depth of character necessary to sustain long-term relationships. This personality type may be encountered more often in the entertainment industry.

Narcissistic Personality Disorder

The primary features of a narcissistic personality disorder are a need for admiration, persistent grandiosity, and a lack of empathy for others. Clients with this disorder have an exaggerated sense of self-importance and accomplishments. They feel that they are superior to others, and should only associate with similar "gifted" individuals. Criteria to meet the diagnosis of narcissistic

personality disorder must include at least five of the following:

1. an exaggerated or grandiose sense of self-importance

2. preoccupation with fantasies of power, wealth, success, and beauty

3. belief of being special and unique, and should only associate with others that are gifted or of high-status

4. a requirement for excessive admiration

5. a sense of entitlement ("owed" things by others)

6. exploitative in interpersonal relationships

7. lacks empathy (unwilling to recognize the feelings and needs of others)

8. envious of others, or believes that others are envious of him

9. arrogant, haughty behaviors or attitudes

Many highly successful clients may display traits that could be considered narcissistic; however, it is only when these traits become maladaptive, inflexible, and cause impairment in important areas of functioning does the diagnosis of a personality disorder apply.

Avoidant Personality Disorder

Clients with avoidant personality disorder display a pattern of social inhibitions, feelings of inadequacy, and hypersensitivity to criticism. They may avoid work or school activities for fear of embarrassment, rejection, or disapproval. Intimate relationships are difficult for these clients. *DSM-IV-TR* diagnostic criteria for this disorder must include at least four of the following:

1. avoids activities that involve significant interpersonal contact for fear of criticism, disapproval, or rejection

2. is unwilling to become involved with people unless certain that they will be liked

3. shows restraint in relationships for fear of shame or ridicule

4. is preoccupied with being criticized or rejected

5. feels inadequate and is inhibited in new situations

6. views self as inferior, socially inept, or unappealing

7. is reluctant to take personal risks or engage in new activities because they might be embarrassing

Avoidant behaviors often begin in childhood with extreme shyness, a tendency to isolate, and fears of strangers or new situations. Behaviors will worsen during adolescence (rather than dissipate as in most people), but there is some evidence that the disorder may become less pronounced with aging.

Dependent Personality Disorder

Individuals with dependent personality disorder demonstrate a pervasive need to be taken care of that leads to clinging and submissive behaviors. These behaviors are designed to elicit caregiving by others. They arise from a self-perception of being unable to function without the help of others. Diagnostic criteria for a dependent personality disorder must include at least five of the following:

1. difficulty making everyday decisions without excess advice and reassurance

2. needs others to take responsibility for most major areas of their life

3. difficulty expressing disagreement with others (fears loss of support or approval)

4. difficulty doing alone (due to a lack of self-confidence)

5. goes to excessive lengths to obtain nurturance and support from others

6. feels uncomfortable or helpless when alone

7. urgently seeks another relationship when one relationship ends

8. is unrealistically preoccupied with fears of being left to take care of self

Clients who have a dependent personality disorder may jump into relationships rapidly, and find themselves in abusive situations from which they are unable to leave because of their extreme fear of being responsible for self-care.

Obsessive-Compulsive Personality Disorder

In contrast to an obsessive-compulsive disorder (OCD), clients with obsessive-compulsive personalities have a preoccupation with orderliness, perfectionism, and mental and interpersonal control at the expense of flexibility, openness, or efficiency. With OCD, clients feel compelled to perform rituals driven by intrusive thoughts in order to reduce or relieve anxiety. Clients with OCD feel driven to check details or follow rules rigidly. They may be oblivious to the annoyance that this can cause others. The perfectionism causes significant dysfunction in the client. *DSM-IV-TR* criteria for obsessive compulsive personality disorder must include at least four of the following:

1. preoccupation with details, rules, lists, order, schedules, or organization

2. perfectionism that interferes with task completion

3. excess devotion to work and productivity to the exclusion of friendships and recreational activities

4. over-conscientious, scrupulous, and inflexible about issues such as ethics, values, or morality

5. unable to discard worn-out or worthless objects — even those without sentimental value

6. reluctant to delegate tasks or work to others

7. miserly-spending style toward self and others (money is viewed as something to be hoarded for catastrophes)

8. shows rigidity and stubbornness

Obsessive-compulsive personality traits can be especially adaptive in certain situations. It is only when the need for control and orderliness become more important than the task or relationship that a personality disorder is diagnosed.

NURSING MANAGEMENT OF THE CLIENT WITH A PERSONALITY DISORDER

Nursing approaches once a personality disorder is identified will vary dependent on the specific needs and concerns of the client. For clients with Cluster-A disorders (paranoid, schizoid, and schizotypal personality disorders), establishing trust and being truthful are important. It is not helpful to challenge ideas or beliefs. Allowing distance from other clients, and not attempting to force social interactions will limit the client's anxiety. Clients demonstrating Cluster-B disorders (antisocial, borderline, histrionic, and narcissistic personality disorders), consistency and a firmer approach may be necessary. There should be a greater emphasis on routines and established rules of the health care setting. The nurse should avoid getting "pulled into" histrionics or staff-splitting behaviors. Positive reinforcement should be provided for socially-acceptable behaviors, while overly dramatic or destructive behaviors should be ignored as much as is safely possible. Cluster-C disorders (dependent, avoidant, and obsessive compulsive personality disorders) may require more nurturance and support by the nurse. Teaching assertiveness skills and relaxation techniques can be helpful. Therapy that focuses on cognitive behavior restructuring should be recommended. Allowing and encouraging the client to make decisions and develop treatment goals will increase a sense of both self-control and empowerment.

BORDERLINE PERSONALITY DISORDER CASE STUDY

Danny is a 32-year-old man with a history of over 10 psychiatric hospitalizations for superficial cuts to his wrists, overdoses, or suicidal threats. He has also been in jail twice: once for a DUI charge, and once for domestic violence. Danny has been in the hospital four times in the past 6 months alone. One year ago, Danny's third wife left him after only 18 months of marriage and filed a restraining order to prevent him from contacting her. Upon examination, Danny tells the nurse that, "life isn't worth living unless you have someone to love you." He also states that "I don't know what I'll do if you make me leave the hospital again." Danny goes on to report that the staff on the previous shift "wouldn't listen to me" and that one of the technicians had threatened to "beat me up if I didn't straighten up and quit lying." Danny feels that the social worker is the only one who really understands him. Since the divorce, Danny has been homeless and staying in shelters. He isn't working "because my ex-wife screwed that up for me" and he has no insurance or source of income. He states his family abused him as a child and, "I won't have anything to do with them." The nurse finds that he has a history of unstable relationships, some of them heterosexual and some of them with same-sex partners. Danny also tends to downplay his substance abuse history stating, "It's really not a problem. I just drink when I'm depressed." Danny's primary admission diagnosis is adjustment disorder with depressed mood, but he is also diagnosed with a borderline personality disorder.

NURSING CARE PLAN

Problem Listing

• Potential for harm to self or to others

- Poor coping strategies to deal with life stressors
- Lack of housing, income, other resources
- Impaired social interactions

Priority Nursing Diagnosis

Potential for harm to self related to impulsivity as evidenced by a history of previous attempts when under severe psychosocial stress.

Long-term Goal

Client will identify and utilize more effective means of dealing with stressors other than harming himself.

Short-term Objectives

1. Client will verbally and in writing contract with staff not to harm himself during the hospital stay.

2. Client will verbalize self-harm urges to staff prior to acting on them.

Nursing Interventions

1. Staff will perform 15-minute safety checks to assess client's well-being.

2. Staff will assist the client in listing five activities to perform to prevent harming himself (for example, journaling, exercising, or calling support hotlines).

3. Staff will assist the client in identifying both precipitants to self-harm behaviors as well as thought processes (cognitive interpretations) of events that led up to those feelings.

EXAM QUESTIONS

CHAPTER 12
Questions 78-84

78. The Power and Control Wheel

    a. divides abuse into different types of controlling behaviors.

    b. demonstrates how domestic violence can lead to death.

    c. explains why men become abusive in relationships.

    d. puts the emphasis of responsibility on the woman.

79. The effects of being in a domestic abuse situation on the partner-victim are to

    a. produce a learned hopelessness and helplessness.

    b. create abnormal relationships in the children.

    c. increase societal costs for incarcerations.

    d. increase feelings of self-control and assertiveness.

80. In childhood sexual abuse

    a. the child may be a willing partner.

    b. the perpetrator is always from a lower-class, home environment.

    c. the non-perpetrating parent is protected from prosecution.

    d. there is always an imbalance in power between perpetrator and victim.

81. The primary feature of a dissociative disorder is

    a. a disruption in consciousness, memory, identity, or perception.

    b. losing blocks of time for days on end.

    c. demonstrating psychotic symptoms unrelated to stressful events.

    d. a sense of detachment or unrealism.

82. Paranoid, schizoid, and schizotypal personality disorders consist of behaviors that appear

    a. anxious and fearful.

    b. manipulative and labile.

    c. dramatic and attention-seeking.

    d. odd or eccentric.

83. Nursing care of Cluster-B personality disorders (antisocial, borderline, histrionic, and narcissistic) should focus on

    a. nurturance and unconditional positive regard.

    b. consistency of routines, rules, and responses to client behaviors.

    c. teaching assertiveness and relaxation techniques.

    d. providing as needed medications for complaints of anxiety.

84. Nursing care that helps the client to set goals, make independent decisions, and learn assertiveness skills is useful for the individual with

    a.   dependent or avoidant personality disorders.

    b.   borderline or histrionic personality disorders.

    c.   antisocial or narcissistic personality disorders.

    d.   paranoid or schizoid personality disorders.

CHAPTER 13

CHILDHOOD DEVELOPMENTAL DISORDERS

CHAPTER OBJECTIVE

At the completion of this chapter, the reader will be able to discuss normal childhood development and recognize cognitive and emotional disorders that arise from disruptions in development.

LEARNING OBJECTIVES

At the end of this chapter, the reader will be able to

1. discuss expected stages of emotional and cognitive development.

2. describe effects of prenatal exposure to drugs and alcohol on the neonate and child.

3. identify the consequences of abuse and neglect for select childhood disorders.

4. recognize and differentiate mental retardation and developmental delay disorders.

5. discuss disorders in learning, communication, and elimination.

NORMAL CHILDHOOD DEVELOPMENT

It is important to have an understanding of normal and expected age-related changes in a child in order to better recognize and treat developmental disorders. In the specialty field of psychiatric nursing, problems in emotional, moral, cognitive, and social development are frequently encountered. In this chapter, several conceptual frameworks with wide acceptance in the field will be utilized to better illustrate these important areas of development.

Sigmund Freud was one of the first clinicians to put forth theories regarding emotional development. Considered somewhat quaint and outdated by many, Freud's theories have the important function of recognizing that needs, desires, and behaviors change as the client matures. Freud believed that changes occur in relationship to a biological drive for the survival and propagation of the species. An overview of his "Stages of Psychosexual Development" is provided in Table 13-1. Stunted development under this model leads to emotional disorders and "neuroses," which are similar to the personality disorders presented in Chapter 12.

In 1950, Erik Erikson developed a theory of emotional development still widely used in nursing and health care settings today. His 8 stages are based on the client's interaction with society. Growth is accomplished through task completion — an inability to obtain a positive outcome at any level will result in a delay of emotional development that may persist late into adulthood. Erikson's "Eight Stages of Psychosocial Development" are covered in Table 13-2. Erikson postulated that if a client is unable to master a particular level (e.g., Trust versus Mistrust) due to poor interpersonal relationships (e.g., childhood sexual abuse), then

TABLE 13-1: FREUD'S STAGES OF PSYCHOSEXUAL DEVELOPMENT

Age of Child	Stage	Primary Focus	Discussion
0-18 months	Oral	Mouth	The subconscious "id" tried to reduce tension by encouraging the child to suck, bite, or chew.
18 months-3 years	Anal	Defecation	Society demands control over impulses and urges resulting in the first conflict with parental figures.
3 years to 5-6 years	Phallic	Genital (penis)	Child becomes infatuated with opposite-sex parent and competitive (jealous) with same-sex parent. Fears castration. Resolves conflict by identifying with same-sex parent and adopting socially-appropriate sex roles.
5-6 years to Puberty	Latency	Cognitive	Skills Stormy periods lessen and energy is devoted to assimilating cultural values and social learning.
Puberty to Adulthood	Genital	Genitals	Energy is directed toward a peer of the opposite sex resulting in mature, adult relationships with the goal of reproduction.

(Wolraich, 1996)

the client is unable to ever fully develop emotionally or complete other developmental tasks (e.g., self-identity, industriousness, or intimacy).

Behavioral learning models are based on the premise that clients grow and learn subsequent to operant conditioning. The best-known behaviorists

TABLE 13-2: ERIKSON'S 8 STAGES OF PSYCHOSOCIAL DEVELOPMENT

Age of Child	Stage	Primary Task	Result of Failure to Complete
0 to 1 year	Trust vs. Mistrust	The development of trust in others. Met by parental love and care taking behaviors.	An inability to develop trust in relationships.
1-3 years	Autonomy vs. Shame/doubt	Developing control of self, including bodily functions.	A sense of insecurity, anxiety, fearfulness
3-5 years	Initiative vs. Guilt	Testing limits. Becoming independent of parents.	A lack of confidence, dependency on others.
5-11 years	Industry vs. Inferiority	Skill development. Rapid learning. Becoming flexible and adaptable.	Overly rigid. Low self-esteem.
11-18 years	Identity vs. Role confusion	Developing a sense of self and how one relates to others. Peer groups.	Confusion over ones place in society. Poor self-concept.
Young adulthood	Intimacy vs. Isolation	Developing love relationships. Learning compromise and giving.	Remaining self-centered. Problems with intimacy.
Adulthood	Generativity vs. Stagnation	Contributing to the greater society. Benefiting future generations.	A sense of hopelessness, or uselessness.
Late adulthood	Ego-integrity vs. Despair	Developing contentment and satisfaction with how life was lived.	Depression. Despair. Feeling of worthlessness.

(Wolraich, 1996)

TABLE 13-3: PIAGET'S STAGES OF COGNITIVE DEVELOPMENT

Age	Stage	Tasks	Comments
Birth to 2 years	Sensorimotor	Increasingly sophisticated responses to the environment.	Child develops symbolic thought representing early language.
2 years to 7 years	Pre-Operational	Trying to make sense of the world.	Thoughts are still rigid and errors in reasoning occur; imagination begins.
7 years to 12 years	Concrete Operational	Internalizing mental operations to learn ideas.	Logical reasoning; less egocentrism; more flexibility; better recognition of social interactions; role-playing.
12 years to Adult	Formal Operational	Applying hypotheses. Formulating ideas.	Abstract thinking begins; ability to use deductive reasoning begins; ability to draw conclusions and project into the future begins.

(Wolraich, 1996)

were Ivan Pavlov and his student B.F. Skinner. Behaviorism states that behaviors that are reinforced positively will be repeated and eventually internalized. Behaviors that are punished or ignored will be extinguished. Acting in a particular way in order to stop a negative reinforcer (e.g., doing homework to stop your parents' nagging) will also cause behaviors to be learned. Operant conditioning principles are widely utilized in school settings, and psychiatric hospitals, and in teaching behavior management techniques to parents.

Vicarious learning is an extension of the behavioral model in that clients can also learn through the process of imitation or modeling. Albert Bandura and R.H. Walters developed a "social learning model" in response to complaints that behaviorism

TABLE 13-4: KOHLBERG'S THEORY OF MORAL DEVELOPMENT

Level	Age	Principles
Preconventional	Substage 1: Birth to preschool age	Children do not consider the interests of others. Actions are based on the avoidance of punishment.
	Substage 2: Preschool to early adolescence	Children become more aware of others and develop ideas of fairness and social exchange.
Conventional	Substage 3: Adolescence	Adolescents begin to appreciate the moral codes of society and become aware of shared feelings and "being good." Requires some "Formal Operational" (Piaget) cognitive development.
	Substage 4: Adolescence	Shifting from relationships between individuals to relationships within groups. Recognition that laws are upheld to avoid the breakdown of society ("law and order" stage).
Postconventional	Substage 5: Young adulthood	The individual recognizes that morality and the law may not be the same; in fact they may conflict with one another. Decisions are made by what is "best" for all concerned.
	Substage 6: Adulthood	Individuals follow self-chosen ethical principles, which may be in conflict with laws. Not all adults develop to this level.

(Wolraich, 1996)

was too passive and did not give credit to the client for being a part of the process. Modeling behaviors after others can help to explain why children grow to behave much like their parents, or why adolescents choose to dress similarly to celebrity musicians or actors (imitation).

Jean Piaget's theory of cognitive development helps us to understand intellectual development. The model stresses that children take an active role in learning and adapting to their environment. It incorporates the concepts of assimilation and accommodation. Assimilation refers to adopting new ideas into existing cognition (e.g., learning that dachshunds, beagles, and terriers are all classes of dogs). Accommodation allows for the learning of new information (e.g., learning that cats are not dogs). Piaget's theory sees intelligence as a process whereby information is assimilated or accommodated at a greater or a lesser degree dependent on the client's existing cognitive abilities. The four stages of cognitive development postulated by Piaget are presented in Table 13-3. Summarized, they represent reflexive responses (birth to age 2), early imagination and use of language (age 2-7), developing concrete ideas and rules (age 7-12), and thinking abstractly using reasoning (age 12 to adulthood). Not all clients will progress to the fourth, or "Formal Operational" stage. Mental retardation or other biological processes may keep a client thinking and reasoning at a level far below chronological expectations.

Lawrence Kohlberg's theory of moral development addresses the manner in which a client develops a sense of right and wrong. He theorized that there are three basic levels of moral reasoning (Table 13-4). Kohlberg's stages are not widely accepted, but they provide an important framework for understanding moral development, particularly in the area of criminal behaviors, frontal lobe injuries, and fetal alcohol syndrome.

PRENATAL ALCOHOL AND DRUG EXPOSURE

One-half to three-quarters of a million children are born each year to mothers who used alcohol or illicit drugs during pregnancy. Little is known about the long-term consequences of prenatal drug exposure on areas of learning, cognitive, and emotional development. Heroin addiction has been associated with increased SIDS (sudden infant death syndrome), which may be related to both the drug itself, and also to the environmental conditions usually encountered by the child. The dramatic increase in the 1980s of cocaine (including "crack") usage contributed to a surge in studies of the immediate effects of cocaine on the newborn. Marijuana is the most commonly used illicit drug during pregnancy, with exposure estimates running from 3% to as high as 20% in some populations. Exposure to alcohol during gestation far exceeds drugs, with alcohol-related birth defects exhibited by upwards of 22,000 children. Legal drugs (such as tobacco) have been associated with low birth weight, premature birth, and intrauterine growth retardation (National Council on Alcoholism and Drug Dependence, Inc., 2001).

Fetal Alcohol Effects

Fetal alcohol effects, and fetal alcohol syndrome by far cause the most dramatic impact on the child. Features of fetal alcohol syndrome have been documented since the 1970s, though vague references can be found in literature going back centuries. There is no reliable way in which to diagnose fetal alcohol effects or fetal alcohol syndrome, other than by a maternal history. In pronounced cases of fetal alcohol syndrome, facial malformations in association with mental retardation provide clues, but in less severe situations there may be no physical changes. Two characteristics appear to be consistent in all children with this disorder: poor impulse control and delayed or stunted moral development. Children with fetal alcohol effects or fetal alcohol syndrome tend to have difficulty in discerning right and wrong, and even when they can verbalize how they "should" behave, their impulsivity and poor insight lead to poor choices. Children with more significant impairments may demonstrate myriad problems including growth retardation, developmental delays, attention-deficit/hyperactivity disorder, small head circumference (microcephaly), a shortened nose, dental abnormalities, cardiac abnormalities, and hearing impairment. Intellectual impairments can range from minimal to severe. Most children born with fetal alcohol effects or fetal alcohol syndrome will require some degree of special education services during the school years.

Cocaine Exposure

Cocaine use during pregnancy can precipitate miscarriage or premature delivery due to a direct positive effect on blood pressure and uterine contractions. Neonates born to cocaine-using women have fewer withdrawal symptoms than seen in opioids; they tend to be jittery, shrill, and to startle easily. Long-term effects are still being studied but early research indicates low birth weight, smaller head circumference, abnormal neonatal behaviors, and a potential for cerebral infarction at birth. Children with a history of cocaine exposure tend to be easily distracted and have a variety of visual-perceptual problems and fine motor difficulties.

Opiate Exposure

Opiate-exposed neonates often have to endure withdrawal symptoms at birth. These can include restlessness, tremulousness, disrupted sleep, poor feeding, stuffy nose, vomiting, diarrhea, a high-pitched cry, fever, irregular breathing, or seizures. Heroin exposure can also cause sneezes, twitches, hiccups, and tearfulness. Symptoms may begin immediately or be delayed up to 4 weeks after delivery, and they will usually resolve at 1 month, but may persist up to 3 months. Growth disturbances, hyperactivity, short attention spans, temper

tantrums, slowed motor development, and impaired visual motor functioning have been reported in children born to opiate-dependent mothers.

Marijuana Exposure

Increased tremulousness, altered visual response patterns to light, and some withdrawal-like crying (irritability), have been noted in children born to women who smoked marijuana heavily during pregnancy. No information is available on long-term consequences of marijuana use during pregnancy.

CHILD ABUSE AND NEGLECT

Although drug and alcohol use during pregnancy is arguably a form of child abuse and neglect, this section will address more direct effects seen in the mental health setting and their impact on child development. Areas to be covered include the failure-to-thrive infant, shaken baby syndrome, Munchausen syndrome by proxy, and reactive attachment disorders. For a more in-depth discussion of childhood sexual abuse, refer to Chapter 12.

Failure-to-thrive

Failure-to-thrive can be defined as a child who fails to gain weight as expected. Causes of failure-to-thrive may include a lack of education in the parents, problems with breastfeeding or formula preparation, problems with digestion, swallowing difficulties, genetic conditions, or neglect. The primary issue in determining neglect is whether reasonable efforts by the parent(s) would allow the child to grow adequately or not, and if the caregivers are making those efforts. Underweight children who grow and flourish in foster care settings are diagnostic of failure-to-thrive neglect. Deprivation of necessary nutrition in an infant and young child can result in inadequate brain development with lifelong consequences, such as poor language or intellectual development.

Shaken Baby Syndrome

Shaken baby syndrome occurs when there is violent shaking of a young child, leading to brain bruising, bleeding, cerebral edema, and other signs of pressure on the brain. Spinal cord injuries may also be present. Almost 90% of shaken babies and young children will demonstrate retinal hemorrhages (in fact, there is little else that causes this physical finding outside of automobile accidents and child abuse). Twenty percent of victims die from complications associated with brain swelling. Long-term consequences include mental retardation, severe developmental delays, visual impairments, and neurological impairments. Perpetrators of shaken baby syndrome are likely to repeat the behaviors. Particularly tragic to parents is the child who dies, or is permanently injured, at the hands of a trusted family member or babysitter.

Munchausen Syndrome by Proxy

Munchausen syndrome by proxy is a rare form of child abuse that consists of the fabrication or production of illness symptoms in a child by the caregiver. The medical symptoms will typically disappear if the child is removed from the environment. Suspicion is aroused when the caregiver presents the child repeatedly for medical care (not injuries) due to a variety of symptoms. Since much of pediatric care is based on the parents' report, children may be diagnosed and treated with numerous medications, have invasive tests and procedures performed, and perhaps even undergo surgery before the diagnosis is suspected. The most common diagnoses seen are chronic vomiting and diarrhea, infections, severe allergies, seizures, and failure-to-thrive. In severe cases, parents have been known to systematically give their children poison, to inject foreign substances into an IV line, or to smear feces in a wound, thereby keeping it infected. Parent behaviors that may be suggestive of this syndrome include highly attentive parents who seem to have excessive medical knowledge; who appear to enjoy the hospital and health care arena and are interested in medical details; who seem to require a great deal of attention from the staff; who demonstrate symptoms similar to the child's; and who appear to be unusually calm, in spite of the serious of the child's illness (Nieves, 2003). Perpetrators of Munchausen syndrome by proxy are not usually in lower socioeconomic groups, in fact the disorder is more prevalent in educated parents with some health care experience. Diagnosis can be confirmed in a hospital setting by hidden cameras in the child's room (most large facilities have rooms set up for this purpose).

Reactive Attachment Disorder

The *DSM-IV-TR* defines reactive attachment disorder as a failure to develop appropriate social-relatedness, usually beginning before age 5, and associated with grossly pathological care. There are two subtypes: inhibited and disinhibited. In the inhibited subtype of reactive attachment disorder, the child demonstrates a pattern of hypervigilant, ambivalent, or highly inhibited behaviors toward caregivers. The child may be resistant to comfort measures, or appear to be watchful or suspicious of others. In the disinhibited type, the child will show diffuse and nondiscriminatory attachments with behaviors such as kissing strangers or climbing into the lap of persons just met. The disorder cannot be accounted for by more pervasive developmental problems (such as retardation or autism). The pathological care history may include a persistent disregard to the child's basic physical or emotional needs, or repeated changes in caregivers that prevent formulation of stable attachments. This disorder is frequently seen in children with a long history of foster home placement, particularly when they have been moved often. Reactive attachment disorder treatment consists of a combination of family therapy and a stable, nurturing, permanent home and caregivers.

MENTAL RETARDATION

Mental retardation is defined by standardized tests that measure intelligence (IQ). A mild mental retardation is an IQ of 55-69. Moderate mental retardation measures from 40-54, severe from 25-39, and profound below 25. Borderline levels (70-80) may be diagnosed as mental retardation, if functioning is poor in important life areas. Cognitive abilities have a significant impact on coping skills, decision-making, and other important areas. There are no consistent behaviors associated with mental retardation; some clients are aggressive or explosive while others may be calm and passive. Clients who have mental retardation have a fourfold risk of developing other mental disorders as compared to the general population. Deficits in communication occur proportionate to the degree of retardation. Causes of mental retardation vary considerably and may include heredity (Down syndrome, fragile X-syndrome), environmental influences (failure-to-thrive), other mental disorders (autism), prenatal problems (alcohol exposure, fetal malnutrition, hypoxia, infections, or trauma), or medical conditions (head injury, lead poisoning). Occasionally, many family members will have greater or lesser degrees of retardation suggesting familial traits, but mental retardation may occur in a child born to parents with normal IQs and no apparent cause as well. Down syndrome clients are encountered frequently in the health care setting and warrant further discussion.

Down Syndrome

Described first in 1866 by Dr. John Langdon Down (but erroneously thought to be related to perinatal tuberculosis), Down syndrome has been seen and treated in health care settings, schools, and residential programs since. Identifying excess material on the 21st chromosome in the deoxyribonucleic acid (DNA) strand makes the diagnosis of Down syndrome. Down syndrome can usually be recognized at birth due to the specific physical characteristics seen:

- Flattened nasal bridge
- Brushfield spots (around the irises)
- Shortened, thick fingers
- Ear abnormalities
- Epicanthal eye folds
- Protruding tongue

TABLE 13-5: MEDICAL PROBLEMS ENCOUNTERED IN DOWN SYNDROME	
System Affected	**Related Disorders**
Neurological	Seizures
	Hypotonia
	Attention-deficit/hyperactivity
	Alzheimer's disease
Musculoskeletal	Joint abnormalities
	Hip instability
	Scoliosis
Cardiovascular	Congenital cardiac lesion
	Mitral valve disease
	AV or ventricular septal defect
	Pulmonary stenosis
Integumentary	Excessive neck skin folds
	Fissured tongue
	Dryness/coarseness/aging
Neurological	Sleep apnea
Hematological	Leukemia
	Polycythemia
Immunological	Increased infections
	Autoimmune disorders
Ear, Nose, Throat	Hearing loss or deafness
	Recurrent otitis media
	Sinus problems and infections
Eye	Brushfield spots (white and yellow nodules circling the iris)
	Conjunctivitis
	Cataracts
Dental	Retained deciduous teeth
	Delayed tooth eruption
	Atypical tooth size or shape
Reproductive	High rate of sterility in men
Gastrointestinal	Anomalies of the GI tract
	Choking problems
	Constipation
	Obesity
Endocrine	Thyroid disease
	Short stature
(Wolraich, 1996)	

Numerous other physical characteristics may also be seen. The degree of mental retardation in Down syndrome can vary from borderline to profound.

Medical problems are common in Down syndrome. Table 13-5 provides an overview of problems frequently seen in the health care setting. Neurological and cardiovascular problems are the most prominent and present the greatest challenge.

Clients who live with Down syndrome can be highly productive members of society. Formerly housed in institutions, they now live independently or with others in a variety of settings. Many clients are employed; some marry and raise families of their own, while others need the support of residential or nursing facilities. Parents of Down syndrome babies should be encouraged to think in terms of their child's future abilities, and not focus on potential disabilities or have lowered expectations.

PERVASIVE DEVELOPMENTAL DISORDERS

A pervasive development disorder is characterized by severe impairment in several areas of development (*DSM-IV-TR*). These disorders are usually evident in the first years of life and may be associated with some degree of mental retardation (though not required). Several types of pervasive development disorders can occur, but all will have some combination of language or communication skill impairment, social interaction impairment, or stereotyped behaviors, interests, or activities. Comorbidity with other psychiatric disorders is extremely high. The two disorders encountered most often in the mental health care setting are autism and Asperger's syndrome.

Autism

Autism is a developmental disorder that is readily recognized early in life. Infants with this disorder are described as aloof or "noncuddly." Repetitive, stereotyped behaviors, such as rocking, spinning or twirling, may be seen. Language acquisition and usage is impaired. Individuals with this disorder may have some degree of mental retardation; some even demonstrate savant characteristics with incredible abilities in music, mathematics, or memorization skills. Hearing problems can occur, which may include deafness or hypersensitivity. Social interactions are dramatically affected — clients with autism have trouble making and keeping friends or they may have no interest in other people at all. Rigid adherence to routines and structure occurs, which may help the clients to maintain some sense of control in their environment.

DSM-IV-TR diagnostic criteria for autism include the following:

1. A total of two or more items from (a) and at least one each from (b) and (c)
   a. Impairment in social interaction
      i. impaired use of nonverbal behaviors such as eye contact, facial expression, body postures, or gestures
      ii. failure to develop age-appropriate peer relationships
      iii. lack of spontaneous seeking to share interests, achievements, or enjoyment with other people
      iv. lack of social or emotional reciprocity
   b. Impairments in communication
      i. delay or lack in a spoken language
      ii. impairment in the ability to initiate or sustain a conversation in the presence of normal speech abilities
      iii. stereotyped and repetitive use of language
      iv. lack of make-believe play or social imitative play appropriate to age

c. Restricted patterns of behavior, interests and activities

  i. preoccupation with abnormally intense or focused interests

  ii. apparently inflexible adherence to specific, nonfunctional routines or rituals

  iii. repetitive motor mannerisms (e.g., hand-flapping)

  iv. preoccupation with parts of objects

2. Delays or abnormal functioning prior to age 3 in at least one of the following areas: social interaction, language used in social communication, or symbolic or imaginative play activities

3. Disorder not better explained by another developmental disorder (e.g., childhood disintegrative disorder or Rett's disorder)

Autism occurs more often in males than females (4-5:1). It is equally distributed across all socioeconomic groups. Prevalence rates indicate that about 10 out of every 10,000 children are born with the disorder, although a study published in 2001 by Chakrabari & Fombonne (in Keltner et al., 2003) increased these numbers to 20 per every 10,000 children (probably because of clearer diagnostic criteria and a more contemporary practice of placing an autism diagnosis as primary, with mental retardation and seizure disorders listed as second or third). Early views on the causes of autism focused on poor parenting and environmental influences. Today it is seen as a neurobiological disorder with diverse physical causes. Autism has recently been linked to early childhood immunizations in a well-published controversy; however, there is no clinical research to support those claims. In many cases, no causative factor for the disorder can be identified. The onset of autism is prior to age 3, but most parents will say that their child "has been this way since birth." There is an increased risk of autistic disorders and other developmental problems among siblings with the disorder (5%). The nature of the impairments in social interaction

may change over time dependent upon the developmental age of the child (*DSM-IV-TR*).

Early identification is essential in order to maximize the child's abilities and provide supportive instruction. Speech therapy, hearing evaluations, occupational therapy, and individualized educational plans may be necessary. A thorough medical examination will help to rule out other disorders (seizure disorders occur in up to 25% of individuals with autism). Concomitant psychiatric disorders often include obsessive-compulsive disorder, attention-deficit/hyperactivity disorder, intermittent explosive disorder, impulse control disorder, and other anxiety or mood disorders. The primary focuses of treatment are to promote the development of social and communication skills, and to improve adaptive living skills to maximum capabilities of the child. Counseling and education for families is also essential.

Asperger's Syndrome

Asperger's syndrome is similar to autism in that the children express developmental problems early in life and there are pronounced social-relatedness problems. In all other ways, it is a markedly different disorder. The essential features of Asperger's syndrome are severe impairment in social interaction along with the development of hyperfocused but restricted patterns of behaviors, interests, or activities. Language development is usually normal if not precocious. Mental retardation rarely occurs. Variability in cognitive and intellectual functioning can occur however, with erratic performances in reading, mathematics, science, music, art, or other abilities. The *DSM-IV-TR* diagnostic criteria for Asperger's syndrome include the following:

1. Impairment in social interaction with at least two of the following:

  a. marked impairment in nonverbal behaviors such as eye-to-eye gaze, facial expression, body postures, or gestures

b. failure to develop peer relationships appropriate to developmental level

c. lack of spontaneous seeking to share enjoyment, interests, or achievements with other people

d. lack of social or emotional reciprocity

2. Restricted repetitive and stereotyped patterns of behavior, interests or activities with at least one of the following:

a. preoccupation with an interest that is abnormal either in intensity or focus

b. inflexible adherence to specific, nonfunctional routines or rituals

c. repetitive motor mannerisms (twisting, rocking, or hand-flapping)

d. preoccupation with parts of objects

There must be clinically significant distress in functioning abilities as well; however, there are no clinically significant delays in language, cognitive development or in age-appropriate self-care skills, curiosity, or adaptive behaviors.

Children with Asperger's syndrome are often acutely aware of their social deficits, but puzzled as to how to behave or respond to others. They can grow into adults who are brilliant scientists, mathematicians, or musicians, but have few friends, which can result in loneliness and low self-esteem. Other psychiatric disorders are also higher in individuals with Asperger's syndrome, most commonly obsessive-compulsive disorders, attention-deficit/hyperactivity disorder, and major depression. Treatment should address any other coexisting disorder. Counseling for clients with Asperger's syndrome is focused on teaching the client more adaptive social skills along with "homework" assignments to practice these skills in a real-world environment.

OTHER DEVELOPMENTAL DISORDERS

A number of different developmental disorders are identified in the *DSM-IV-TR* including academic-based disorders (reading, writing, and arithmetic), communication disorders, disorders of feeding in early childhood, and elimination disorders. For the purpose of simplicity, these will be grouped into broad categories for discussion.

Reading, Writing, and Arithmetic Disorders

Disorders that involve reading, written words, or understanding mathematical concepts are frequently encountered in the academic setting (as opposed to the psychiatric). A learning disorder is diagnosed when an client's achievement on standardized tests is substantially below that expected for age, schooling, and level of intelligence. The learning problems must also interfere with academic achievement or daily living activities that require those skills (such as filling out job applications or balancing a checkbook in an adult, or learning to count money in a child). Other conditions such as generalized mental retardation, visual problems, or hearing loss must be ruled out. Reading disorders are diagnosed 60-80% of the time in males, with a prevalence of 4% of all school-age children. Diagnosis usually does not occur until 1st grade when it becomes more readily apparent. Reading disorders can take a variety of forms that may include dyslexia (reversing letters or words), visual-perceptual problems, and reading comprehension problems. Mathematics disorders are identified later (2nd or 3rd) grade because of the more advanced skills required at those ages. Mathematics disorders are less common, occurring in about 1% of school-age children. Disorders of written expression (writing) are difficult to separate from other learning disorders, as writing skills are dependent upon a complex interaction between reading and comprehension, and motor coordination. The diagnosis is not given if the only problem noted is sloppy or poor handwriting. Tasks in which a child is asked to copy, write to dictation, or write spontaneously will better uncover this disorder. School testing and an individualized educational plan (IEP) are usually necessary for children with these disorders.

Language and Communication Disorders

Communication disorders consist of both expressive and receptive language disorders, phonological disorder, and stuttering. Expressive language disorders require that the child scores lower than expected on standardized tests that measure language development. Frequently, children will demonstrate word-finding or vocabulary errors, a limited range of vocabulary, a limited amount of speech, difficulty acquiring new words, simplified or shortened sentences, use of unusual word order, omissions of parts of sentences and a slow rate of language development that is not consistent with their IQ. If the child also has a sensory deficit, severe environmental deprivation, or mental retardation, then the language delay must be more than that which would be expected for that disorder. Schoolwork suffers and grades are low in reading, language, and spelling due to the child's inability to express himself verbally or in writing. A mixed receptive-expressive language disorder is one in which standardized scores in both expressive and receptive language abilities are lower than would be expected. With this disorder, expressive language problems are always present, but the child also demonstrates difficulties in understanding language. Problems understanding words, sentences, or phrases may exist. In mild cases, understanding complicated language structure may be all that is impaired. In severe cases, understanding basic vocabulary, discriminating sounds, associating sounds with symbols, storage, recall, and sequencing may all be affected. Because expressive abilities always rely on perception and understanding, a pure receptive language disorder does not exist (as may be seen in adults with cerebral vascular accidents).

A phonological disorder (formerly called a developmental articulation disorder) is a failure to use developmentally expected speech sounds. Common errors seen are mispronunciations of letters (*r, th, ch*) or substitutions of one sound for another (e.g., *t* for *k*). Lisping (*th* for *s*) is relatively common. Phonological development problems are more prominent in males than in females, and present in about 2% of the population. Environmental factors should be considered when assessing a child's speech (learned patterns). About three-quarters of affected children spontaneously remit by age 6. Speech therapy through the school system may be indicated for enduring problems.

Stuttering differs from phonological problems in that the pronunciation of the letters and words is not impaired, but there is a disturbance in the fluency and time patterning of the speech. There may be frequent repetitions of prolongations of sounds, syllables or words. Blocking (silences between words), broken words (pauses within a word), word substitutions, or other disturbances may be seen. The extent and intensity of the disturbance varies between situations and is often more severe when the client is feeling under pressure or anxious. Stuttering may be absent when reading aloud, singing, or talking to pets or toys. Motor movements, such as eye-blinking or head-jerking, may accompany stuttering. It is three times higher in males than in females, and occurs in 1% of children prior to puberty (0.8% post pubescent). Speech therapy and relaxation counseling can help clients to live with the disorder.

PICA

Several disorders may occur in young children that affect eating and feeding behaviors, which may in turn have a negative impact on development. These are differentiated from anorexia nervosa and bulimia nervosa in that there is no perception of being overweight or a desire to lose weight, as seen in those disorders. Of most clinical interest is the unusual eating of nonnutritive substances on a persistent basis for at least 1 month known as pica. Very young children may eat paint (which can contain lead), plaster, hair, string, or cloth. Older children may consume sand, insects, leaves, pebbles, or animal dropping. Adolescents tend to eat clay, soil or starch. Pica is also found in pregnant women, and has been associated with iron deficiencies in that population. To be diagnosed as a disorder, the behavior may not be a part of a culturally sanctioned practice (some countries regularly encourage the consumption of clay with meat). Children with pica do not have any particular aversions to eating "normal" food as well. Pica is frequently associated with mental retardation and pervasive developmental disorders, although it may occur in other children as well. Although there are some reports of vitamin or other nutrient deficiencies, these are not consistent and a cause cannot always be found. Complications of pica include poisoning, bowel obstruction, intestinal perforations, or infections (e.g., parasitic). Some substances are harmless, and the behavior can be ignored. In other cases, increased supervision of the child may be necessary.

ELIMINATION DISORDERS

Two types of elimination disorders are seen in children: encopresis and enuresis. To be diagnosed as a psychiatric or behavioral disturbance, medical causes must first be ruled out. The essential feature of encopresis is the passing of feces (either voluntarily or involuntarily) into inappropriate places (clothing, closets, floor, or toy box). The behavior must occur at least once a month for 3 months or more, and the child must be over the age

of four. Encopresis is often the result of constipation or impaction, which may be due to psychological stress (anxiety, fear, defiance), or illnesses such as dehydration. Painful stool passage will predispose the child to avoidance behavior, which will in turn increase the withholding and cause constipation. Occasionally a child is incontinent of liquid, runny stools secondary to fecal retention. Encopresis is seen in many children, but its association to severe distress (such as that experienced following sexual abuse) warrants close attention when obtaining a nursing history. Encopresis can be socially devastating to a child, resulting in repeated embarrassment and ostracizing by other children.

Treatment for encopresis involves bowel-retraining programs. The child is usually put on a daily laxative (such as mineral oil) and may also be given a fiber supplement daily. Educate the parents about high-fiber diets that include fruit juices (especially apple and grape), whole fruits, vegetables, and whole grain cereals. Also teach the parents to have their child sit on the toilet on a regular basis, usually right after breakfast, and sit without straining for several minutes (if necessary, the child should be taken to the toilet every 4 hours until successful, but not left sitting more than 5 or 6 minutes each time). Extra clean clothes should be taken to the school and left at the health aid's office. Alerting the health aid or school nurse and classroom teacher of the problem may help to diminish some of the stigma associated with encopresis.

Enuresis is the involuntary (or voluntary) passage of urine at inappropriate times or in inappropriate places. Enuresis is subdivided into "nocturnal only," "diurnal only," and "both nocturnal and diurnal" subtypes. Criteria to diagnose enuresis require that the "accidents" occur at least twice a week for 3 months or more in a child who is at least age 5. The amount of impairment associated with enuresis is dependent upon the age, subtype and how it impacts on peer relationships. A 6-year-old who wets the bed every night is not as devastating as is a 12-year-old who wants to stay over at a friend's home or go camping. Prevalence rates for enuresis are relatively high: 5-10% of all children under the age of 10. There is a significant familial component with 75% of children having a family member with a history of the disorder. Enuresis is more likely in children with attention-deficit/hyperactivity disorder, developmental delays, sleep disorders, or urinary tract infections. Enuresis is less related to psychological distress than is encopresis.

Once medical causes are ruled-out, treatment of enuresis is usually a combination of medications and behavior modification. Medications used include DDAVP® (desmopressin), a synthetic antidiuretic hormone or imipramine (Tofranil®), a tricyclic antidepressant. Both are administered at bedtime. DDAVP is available orally (doses are usually 0.1-0.3 mg) or in a nasal spray (1 spray in each nostril). Imipramine is only available orally and is usually dosed at 10 mg. Doses higher than 20 mg place the child at risk for slowed cardiac conduction and an electrocardiogram (EKG) reading is advised. Two types of behavior management are useful for treating enuresis. In the first, parents may purchase a pad that sets off an alarm when it becomes wet. The alarm is designed to wake the child, prompting a visit to the toilet. Hopefully, the child will eventually become conditioned to waking at that same time every night. The second method requires that parents set an alarm clock and check on the child at increasingly earlier hours nightly until they find the point at which the bed becomes wet during the night. They then must wake the child immediately prior to that "wetting time" every night and escort the child to the bathroom, until the child wakes up automatically. It is always prudent to restrict fluids within an hour of bedtime, and to ask the child to urinate before retiring. Using pull-up diapers at night can be acceptable in young children, but they may be emotionally traumatic for the older child (in addition, they tend to give "permission" for wetting behaviors). Diurnal, or daytime, wetting is best treated by toileting routines of escorting (or sending) the child to the bathroom every 2-3 hours, including during the school day.

DEVELOPMENTAL DISORDER CASE STUDY

Matthew is an 8-year-old boy with autistic disorder who presents in the health care facility for an increase in aggressive behaviors. His mother reports that he was first recognized as autistic at age 3. He has difficulty relating to others, and prefers to play alone with his toy cars (stacking them and twirling their wheels), which he can do for hours. Lately, he has started to lick the backs of his hands repetitively and they are red and chapped. Whenever family members or schoolteachers ask him to stop playing or licking and attend to tasks-at-hand (such as schoolwork or a family meal), he starts to yell and rock back and forth. If he is touched, he strikes out violently against anyone he can reach. Matthew has difficulty in using language to express his needs, and at times he doesn't seem to understand what is being asked of him. In addition to the autism diagnosis, academic testing has revealed an IQ of 72. Medical findings are as follows: 4'10", 75 lb, BP 110/58, heart rate 110; hands are chapped and reddened; nails are bitten to the quick; nocturnal enuresis 4-5 nights out of 7; rare diurnal enuresis; rare encopresis; sleep is decreased with an onset of 11 p.m. and awake by 5 a.m. daily; appetite is erratic; increased motor activity and impulsive striking out.

Matthew is placed on Luvox® 25 mg at bedtime to be titrated to 50 mg at bedtime (h.s.) in 1 week and DDAVP nasal spray bilateral nares (h.s.). A toileting routine was also discussed with his parents to facilitate in his staying dry at night.

NURSING CARE PLAN

Problem Listing

- Bedwetting 4 or 5 nights out of 7
- Sleep onset problems
- Red, chapped hands (potential for infection)
- Impulsive, aggressive behaviors
- Inflexibility with changes in routines

Priority Nursing Diagnosis

Risk for violence directed toward others related to poor impulse control as evidenced by striking out at caregivers when redirected.

Long-term Goal

Client will learn alternative ways to communicate his needs without resorting to aggression.

Short-term Objectives

1. Client will not strike out more than once a month.

2. Client will demonstrate "personal time-outs" when feeling upset prior to striking out.

Nursing Interventions

1. Educate parents to recognize the four stages of crisis escalation:

   a. Trigger (events that precipitate acting-out)

   b. Escalation (behaviors that indicate increasing tension)

   c. Acting-out (striking out or destructive behaviors)

   d. De-escalation (calming down)

2. Educate parents as to means of dealing with each stage as it occurs:

   a. Trigger — identify precipitants then work to reduce or eliminate them

   b. Escalation — recognize signs of tension (e.g., pacing or rocking), then help child to redirect his energy or to take a personal time-out

   c. Acting-out — place child in safe time-out area; may use as needed medications if they are available

   d. De-escalation — talk with child about what led to time-out (e.g., "In this family we don't hit other people," reassure child, for example, "You're a good boy and we love you.")

3. Ask parents to log acting-out behaviors for one week, then help them to analyze the triggers, how they responded to signs of escalation and acting-out, and how the process of de-escalation occurred.

4. Educate parents in ways to help their child transition between activities in order to reduce stress-responses (e.g., giving 5-minute warnings, getting eye contact prior to giving directions, and asking him to repeat directions.)

CHAPTER 13
Questions 85-92

85. The stage of growth and development entitled "Identity versus Role Confusion" usually emerges in

    a. early childhood.

    b. adolescence.

    c. young adulthood.

    d. old age.

86. Piaget's stage of formal operational thought requires

    a. reflexive and interactive play.

    b. cause-and-effect relationships.

    c. abstract thinking and reasoning abilities.

    d. social reciprocity.

87. A jittery, shrill baby that startles easily may have been exposed prenatally to

    a. heroin.

    b. cocaine.

    c. ecstasy.

    d. marijuana.

88. Signs of heroin withdrawal in a neonate include

    a. listlessness, fatigue, and poor feeding.

    b. hypotonia and seizures.

    c. tremulousness, sneezes, and a high-pitched cry.

    d. irritability and light sensitivity.

89. Reactive attachment disorder is a failure to develop appropriate social relatedness associated with

    a. grossly pathological care.

    b. neurological delays.

    c. educational deprivation.

    d. sensory deprivation problems.

90. Diagnostic criteria for autism will include impairments in

    a. social interaction and communication.

    b. thought processes and intelligence.

    c. emotional expression and anger control.

    d. reading and arithmetic abilities.

91. A failure to use developmentally expected speech sounds is a(n)

    a. expressive language disorder.

    b. receptive language disorder.

    c. phonological disorder.

    d. stuttering disorder.

92. Encopresis is most often related to

    a. constipation brought about by psychological stress.

    b. poor sphincter control.

    c. defiance and a desire to soil on others.

    d. severe and profound developmental delays.

CHAPTER 14

DISRUPTIVE BEHAVIOR AND TOURETTE'S DISORDER

CHAPTER OBJECTIVE

At the completion of this chapter, the reader will be able to describe disruptive behavior disorders and Tourette's disorder, and discuss relevant treatments.

LEARNING OBJECTIVES

At the end of this chapter, the reader will be able to

1. describe the symptoms and management of Attention-Deficit/Hyperactivity Disorder (ADHD)

2. discuss medication interventions and nursing management of the child with ADHD.

3. differentiate ADHD from oppositional defiant disorder and conduct disorder.

4. recognize motor and vocal tics and their relationship to Tourette's disorder.

ATTENTION-DEFICIT/ HYPERACTIVITY DISORDER

Attention-Deficit/Hyperactivity Disorder (ADHD) is the most frequently encountered psychiatric diagnosis in children with prevalence rates around 4%. The core features of ADHD have been described in the literature since the 1930s,

although terminology has changed over time. Early diagnoses were minimal brain damage and minimal brain dysfunction, since it was felt that ADHD symptoms were similar to behaviors seen in clients with central nervous system (CNS) injuries. In the 1950s the diagnosis was changed to hyperactive child syndrome. The *DSM-II* altered the diagnosis to be hyperkinetic reaction of childhood in 1968, which constituted the prevailing standard until 1980. The *DSM-III* first recognized that ADHD was a disorder of attention as well as hyperactivity. In 1984, the *DSM-IV* further described ADHD utilizing the subtypes of "with hyperactivity," "without hyperactivity," and "combined presentation" (Mick, 2002).

Much of the difficulty in diagnosing ADHD arises out of the fact that many of its symptoms are developmentally appropriate in certain contexts. For example, 4-year-old children are talkative, impulsive, and extremely active. A diagnosis of ADHD can only be made when the symptoms are determined to be at a level that is greater than expected for the average child. *DSM-IV-TR* criteria for diagnosing ADHD are as follows:

1. Either (a) or (b)

   a. Six (or more) of the following symptoms of inattention have been present for at least 6 months at a degree that is maladaptive and developmentally inconsistent:

      i. fails to give close attention to details

or makes careless mistakes in work or other activities

ii. has difficulty sustaining attention during tasks or play activities

iii. does not seem to listen when spoken to directly

iv. does not follow through on instructions and fails to finish tasks once started

v. has difficulty in organizing tasks or activities

vi. avoids, dislikes, or is reluctant to engage in tasks that require mental effort (such as schoolwork)

vii. loses things necessary for activities or tasks

viii. is easily distracted by external stimuli

ix. is often forgetful in daily activities

b. Six or more of the following symptoms of hyperactivity-impulsivity have persisted for at least 6 months at a level that is maladaptive:

i. fidgets with hands or feet or squirms in seat

ii. leaves the seat in the classroom or other situations where it is inappropriate (e.g., church, dinner table)

iii. runs about or climbs excessively in inappropriate situations

iv. has difficulty playing or engaging in leisure activities quietly

v. is often "on the go" or acts as if "driven by a motor"

vi. often talks excessively

vii. often blurts out answers before questions have been completed

viii. has difficulty taking turns

ix. often interrupts or intrudes on others

2. Some symptoms have to be present prior to age 7

3. Some form of impairment from the symptoms presenting in two or more settings (e.g., home and school, home and grandparents home)

4. Symptoms clearly interfering with social and family relationships, academic performance, or occupational functioning

5. Symptoms cannot be better accounted for by another disorder

The subtypes of ADHD are based on whether both (a) and (b) were met or not. ADHD, predominately inattentive type is diagnosed when only criterion (a) is met; ADHD, predominately hyperactive-impulsive type is diagnosed when only criterion (b) is met; and ADHD, combined type is diagnosed when at least 6 symptoms are present from both (a) and (b).

Features that are not part of the diagnostic criteria but are certainly associated with ADHD will vary with developmental age and may include low frustration tolerance, temper outbursts (common), bossiness, stubbornness, demanding, mood lability, depressed moods, poor peer interactions, and low self-esteem. Peers may reject or refuse to play with children with ADHD. Academic achievement is usually markedly impaired, in spite of normal or above normal intellectual capabilities. This often contributes to a great deal of conflict between the child and the parents leading to strained family dynamics. The hyperactive and impulsive symptoms often cause the child to get into trouble at school or in other settings. Lost recess time, in-school suspensions, frequent visits to the principal's office, or even suspensions and expulsions may result, which serve to further interrupt the learning process. Individuals with ADHD, predominately inattentive type have few behavior problems, but they tend to be withdrawn, socially passive, and neglected by peers.

Almost half of the children diagnosed with ADHD (hyperactive-impulsive or combined types)

also have oppositional or defiant behaviors, or conduct disorders. This co-occurrence is significantly higher for ADHD than for other psychiatric disorders. Almost one-third of children with ADHD will have another concomitant disorder. The most common diagnoses reported are anxiety disorders, mood disorders (both major depression and bipolar disorder), learning disorders or communication disorders (*DSM-IV-TR*).

Causes of ADHD are not known. It has been found to be more common among first-degree biological relatives, lending credibility to genetic factors. In some children, there may be a history of child abuse or neglect, lead or other toxin exposures, brain infections, prenatal drug or alcohol exposure, or mental retardation. Prematurity and low birth weights have been associated with ADHD, though there is no research evidence to support this claim.

There are no laboratory tests or other physical findings that will diagnose or suggest ADHD. Physical examinations should be completed to rule-out other causes of overactivity (e.g., thyroid disease) or mood lability (e.g., type I diabetes mellitus). Administering structured assessments to parents, select teachers, and other involved adults is done in order to evaluate for the disorder. Direct observations are also helpful, but children with ADHD are frequently able to behave well or pay attention for short periods of time and during one-on-one appointments (such as in an office setting). Parent history is the best source of diagnostic information. Other psychiatric disorders such as major depression or childhood-onset schizophrenia may mimic the inattentive components of ADHD. Table 14-1 provides a comparison of some of the more common symptoms of these disorders seen in children.

ADHD is two to three times more common in males than in females, although the predominately inattentive type has fewer gender distinctions. Most parents first observe ADHD symptoms when their child is a toddler, but occasionally parents will report that even as an infant the child was restless and "squirmy," or a "difficult baby." The symptoms of ADHD (in particular the hyperactivity criteria) tend to stabilize during adolescence and may remit in young adulthood in a majority of the cases. Some ADHD symptomatology may persist into adulthood and cause problems with job stability, financial security, and relationships with significant others.

TABLE 14-1: SYMPTOMS OF ADHD AND OTHER DISORDERS

Disorder	Hyperactivity or Restlessness	Impulsivity	Decreased Attention Span or Poor Concentration	Decreased Sleep	Appetite Changes	Cognitive Impairments (hallucinations, delusions, disorganized thoughts)	Mood Changes (sadness, grouchiness, irritability, anxiety)	Physical Complaints (GI upset, headaches)
ADHD Combined	Yes	Yes	Yes	Yes	No	No	Not usually	No
ADHD Inattentive	No	No	Yes	No	No	No	Not usually	No
ADHD Hyper-Imp.	Yes	Yes	No	Yes	No	No	Not usually	No
Major Depression	May occur	Not likely	Yes	Yes	Yes	May occur	Yes	May occur
Anxiety Disorders	Yes	Not likely	Yes	No	Yes	No	Yes	Yes
Childhood Schizophrenia	Not likely	May occur	Yes	No	No	Yes	No	Not likely

TREATMENT INTERVENTIONS FOR ADHD

Parent Education

Educating the parents becomes a priority once a diagnosis of ADHD is established; parents need to understand that ADHD is believed to be related to chemical and neurological alterations in the brain, and not a result of poor parenting practices. ADHD is a well-publicized disorder and parents may have preconceived ideas about the diagnosis based on both accurate and inaccurate media reports and the opinions of family members. Additionally, ADHD is a disorder of deficits and not one of noncompliance; that is to say that children with the disorder are not intentionally hyperactive or inattentive; rather they are as much at a loss to understand why they behave in such ways as are the adults in their lives. Repeatedly punishing a child for impulsive behaviors will succeed only in frustrating both the child and the parent, and may result in significant self-esteem problems as well. Basically, children with ADHD want to do well and to please their parents and teachers, but they are unable to force themselves to be asymptomatic (in many ways this is similar to asking an epileptic child to stop having seizures merely by force of will power). Parents also have a responsibility to learn as much as possible about the disorder in order to serve as an advocate with the school systems and, in severe cases, with various social service or government agencies. Parent support groups are an invaluable way in which parents can receive ongoing education and interactions with other parents who may be having similar problems. Children and Adults with Attention Deficit Disorders (CHADD) is a support and advocacy program that also functions as a legislative watchdog for educational bills that may have a significant impact on the education of a child with ADHD. Their Web site, located at www.chadd.org, contains a wealth of information for parents and adults with ADHD.

Behavior Management

A second and equally important component of ADHD treatment is training parents in behavior management. Utilizing basic techniques of both positive and negative reinforcers, negative consequences, and ignoring some behaviors, parents can motivate their children to function at a maximum level. Clients with ADHD often do not feel in control of themselves. Implementing behavior management techniques improves a sense of self-control that contributes to feeling proud of one's accomplishments and improved self-esteem. Parents should be assisted in identifying target behaviors that need modification, such as having tantrums, acting-up in the classroom, or refusing to do homework. Vague and ill-defined problems (e.g., "being bad" or "poor attitude") should be avoided. Once problem behaviors are identified, the parent and child together determine positive reinforcers that will be awarded the child on a daily or weekly basis when the problem behaviors are avoided. Rewards have to be meaningful to the child; for example, monetary rewards may not be as intrinsically rewarding as special favors such as a later bedtime or a trip to the ice cream parlor. Conversely, the parent and child need to have negative consequences for the continuance of the problematic behavior. Negative consequences should be clear, concise and nonnegotiable; being "grounded" from television or videogames, or having an early bedtime are good choices for the younger child. Suspending phone privileges or preventing visits with friends are more appropriate for the adolescent. Negative reinforcement refers to the removal of a noxious stimuli when a problem behavior improves; for example, keeping the child under continuous supervision during homework is a negative reinforcer that is removed once the homework is completed or the child learns to work independently. Some behaviors also can be ignored. Behaviors that are essentially harmless (e.g., whining or nonphysical tantrums) may be inadvertently positively reinforced when a parent responds to the behavior. Ignoring the behavior prevents its reinforcement and it will eventually extinguish. Naturally, behaviors that could potentially be harmful to the client or others will have to be dealt with immediately.

Time-outs are an effective means of managing acting-out behaviors. The purpose of a time-out is to assist children in learning to calm themselves, and it should not be perceived as a punishment. Timing is crucial — the time-out should begin immediately when acting-out occurs (not 4 hours later or "when your father gets home") and it should end when the child is calm and rational. During a time-out, the child should not receive any form of attention from the parent(s) including attempts to "make the child understand." Attention itself will serve as a positive reinforcer. As soon as the time-out is over, the parent should reconnect with the child through eye contact and praise the child for calming down; then the parent and child need to discuss the events that led up to the time-out and how they might be avoided in the future. For a young child this may be as simple as the statement, *"Johnny, you're a good little boy and I love you very much. In this family we don't hit and call names."* Older children can be asked to verbalize or write down the problem, why it occurred, and what could have been done differently. Personal time-outs are a useful tool to teach a child. The child in recognition of increasing tension initiates a personal time-out. The "rules" for a personal time-out are that the child may state *"I need a break"* and leave the situation without being pursued by the parent or sibling involved. When sufficiently calm, the child can return to the situation to discuss it more rationally. Clinicians vary in opinions on where a time-out should be taken. A chair in the busiest room of the house is never a good idea. Because a time-out is a chance to learn self-control and calm down, playing quietly with toys can be productive; therefore, sending a child to his bedroom is probably the best option. It also communicates a message to the child that undesirable behaviors will not be tolerated in the general family environment.

Environmental structure and predictability are also very important for children with ADHD, perhaps because the child feels so out of control himself. Transitions (changing from one activity to another) are extremely difficult for children with ADHD. The parents should make as much effort as possible to keep household routines consistent; getting up, eating meals, doing homework, allowing for play time, and going to bed at the same time every day will assist in this process. Parents can expect children with ADHD to have some worsening in behavior after weekends, extended vacations, or visitation with noncustodial parents. Children will also act-out more at school when regular classroom teachers are gone and substitutes are in their place.

Educational Interventions

Although intellect is not usually a problem, children with ADHD often require individualized educational plans under the category of emotional handicap. Teachers and schools may need to make special accommodations for the child including such things as extra study-hall time, in-class tutors, or physical rearrangements of the classroom (to reduce opportunities for distraction). Parents have to be active in the learning process and supervise homework assignments vigilantly. Frequently, homework scores and grades are used to determine the effectiveness of treatment interventions.

MEDICATION INTERVENTIONS FOR ADHD

Medications have been used for ADHD since the 1950s when methylphenidate (Ritalin®) was first introduced. It is important to explain to parents that medications do not "cure" ADHD; rather they treat the symptoms of the disorder by altering neurotransmitters, primarily dopamine. The same medications are used regardless of the ADHD subtype. Five broad categories of medications are in common usage: stimulants, alpha-adrenergics, norepinephrine-reuptake inhibitors, antipsychotics, and certain antidepressants. An

overview of ADHD medications is provided in Table 14-2.

Stimulants

Stimulants are highly treatment-effective for improving focus, concentration, attention span, and reducing distractibility and overactivity. They work by delaying the release of dopamine from the neurotransmitters in the brain, thus slowing or regulating chemical conduction at the neuron level. Stimulants are chemically in the classification of amphetamines or amphetamine-like agents. Some children tolerate one type of stimulant better than another. Young children may do better with shorter acting agents (Focalin®, Ritalin®, Adderall®) while older children and adolescents usually prefer a

TABLE 14-2: MEDICATIONS TO TREAT ATTENTION-DEFICIT/HYPERACTIVITY DISORDER

Category	Generic Name	Trade Name	Sedation	Weight Gain	Ortho. BP risk	Insomnia	GI Upset	Dry Mouth, Constipation	Comments
Stimulants (related to Amphetamines)	methylphenidate	Ritalin® Ritalin SR®	—	—	—	+++	+++	+	First ADHD med. developed Short duration at 3-4 hr May induce tic disorder
	dexmethylphenidate	Focalin®	—	—	—	++	++	+	More specific than Ritalin
	methylphenidate	Metadate ER®, Metadate CD®	—	—	—	++	++	+	Duration of 6-8 hr Good for young school-age child
	methylphenidate	Concerta®	—	—	—	+++	++	+	Duration of 12 hr
	dextroamphetamine	Dexedrine®	—	—	—	++	++	+	Duration of 4-6 hr
	Combination of dextroamphetamine sulfate & saccharate, and amphetamine sulfate & aspartate	Adderall® Adderall XR®	—	—	—	+++	++	+	Duration of 4-6 hr for immediate release, 12 hr for XR. Sprinkle tablets for children that can't swallow pills/capsules.
	pemoline	Cylert®	—	—	—	++	++	+	Black Box warning: Liver failure
Norepinephrine Reuptake Inhibitor	atomoxetine	Strattera®	++	+	—	+	++	+	New in 2003. Once-a-day dosing; takes 4 weeks to be fully effective
Alpha-adrenergics	clonidine	Catapres® Catapres TTS®	+++	—	+++	—	—	—	Treats hyper & impulsive sxs. Very sedating. Good as an h.s. adjunct. Suppresses motor tics.
	guanfacine	Tenex®	++	—	+++	—	—	—	Treats tics; good for impulsivity
Antidepressants	buproprion	Wellbutrin® Wellbutrin SR®	—	—	—	+	—	—	Acts on dopamine system Better for adolescents or adults with ADHD; no abuse potential.
	imipramine	Tofranil®	+++	++	++	—	—	+++	Primary use is enuresis. Cardiac conduction delays are possible.
	venlafaxine	Effexor XR®	—	+	—	—	+	+	Useful in ADHD + Depression
Antipsychotics	risperidone	Risperdal®	++	++	+	—	—	+++	Good for aggressive sxs +ADHD
	olanzapine	Zyprexa®	+++	+++	—	—	—	++	Good for bipolar sxs + ADHD
	quetiapine	Seroquel®	+++	++	+	—	—	++	Good as HS sleeper in ADHD

+++ High ++ Moderate + Low — Negligible

long-acting medicine (Adderall XR®, Concerta®, Metadate CD®). Stimulant medications work within 15-20 minutes, and are completely metabolized and eliminated by the body in the same day. They provide flexibility in dosing with some parents choosing to utilize them on school days only. Side effects to stimulant medications at therapeutic doses may include jitteriness, gastrointestinal (GI) upset, decreased appetite, and insomnia. Weight loss can be significant in some children; weight should be checked at each follow-up appointment or at least every 3 months. Indications that the medication is dosed too high are cognitive dulling, a flattened affect, or agitation and mood lability. Overdosage can result in toxicity symptoms (hallucinations, tachycardia, cardiac arrhythmias). Occasionally children may develop motor tics at any dosage. Formerly, tic development was an indication to discontinue or change the medication. Today clinicians are not as concerned about motor tics as they tend to resolve spontaneously by age 10-12. Serum levels are not necessary when utilizing stimulant medications — dosages are determined based on clinical response and side effects.

Alpha-adrenergics

Alpha-adrenergics are medications that have an off-label use in treating the overactivity, hyperarousal, and impulsivity associated with ADHD, combined and hyperactive-impulsive types. They do little to help with focus or concentration. Alpha-adrenergics are more commonly used as antihypertensives in adults. They appear to work by reducing norepinephrine levels in primarily the frontal cortex of the brain. Two medications are prescribed: guanfacine (Tenex®) and clonidine (Catapres®, Catapres TTS® Transdermal). Side effects to these medications include drowsiness or sedation, and dizziness. Doses should be titrated slowly, and BP checks should be done on follow-up appointments. Children rarely have blood pressure drops on the dosages used for ADHD. There are no long-acting

forms of these medications. Dosing is usually required three to four times per day (t.i.d.-q.i.d.). Alpha-adrenergics may be prescribed in combination with stimulants. They are also effective in suppressing motor tic activity.

Norepinephrine-reuptake inhibitor

A new medication, atomoxetine (Strattera®) was launched in 2003 to treat ADHD in a different way. Strattera® is a norepinephrine-reuptake inhibitor, which means that it slows down the transmission of norepinephrine through the neuronal pathways. It is highly effective in reducing hyperactive-impulsive symptoms, and moderately effective in improving the inattention symptoms. It may also be useful for modulating the moodiness and irritability experienced by some children. Strattera® is not immediately effective; it requires a titration over 4-5 days, then it takes 2-4 weeks to achieve steady state. Dosing is based on the weight of the child. Common side effects reported to date include GI upset and drowsiness. It may be dosed once a day at bedtime, which makes it useful for children who have difficulty in settling down to sleep. Occasionally it can cause CNS activation and should be dosed in the morning. Some clinicians are now utilizing Strattera® at night and a low-dose stimulant medication in the morning.

Atypical Antipsychotics

Another alternative is to utilize new-generation "atypical" antipsychotics in children with ADHD. Of these, risperidone (Risperdal®) has the most literature available, but Zyprexa® and Seroquel® are also used quite frequently. The newest agents, Geodon® and Abilify™, are not yet in common practice. Antipsychotics work by blocking dopamine release in the neurons. These medications are particularly useful for children that have a high level of aggression and mood instability. Side effects are reviewed extensively in Chapter 4; the most common ones are sedation, increased appetite and tremors at high doses. Weight gain can be pronounced in some children and it should be monitored at follow-up appointments. Extrapyramidal syndrome side effects and signs of tardive dyskinesia should be evaluated and the dose lowered or weaned off if they are detected. Risperdal® may also elevate prolactin levels and cause dysmenorrhea or breast milk production in the adolescent. Its effects on puberty and menarche are not known.

Antidepressants

Antidepressants have some usefulness in ADHD treatment. Tricyclic antidepressants (TCAs), such as Tofranil®, Norpramin®, have been shown to be helpful, probably due to their potent norepinephrine effects. TCAs have to be used with caution, however, because of concerns over cardiac conduction delays. Serum monitoring and electrocardiograms (EKGs) are indicated. Selective serotonin reuptake inhibitors (SSRIs) do not demonstrate any significant positive effects on ADHD. They are quite useful, however, for children with concomitant depression or anxiety disorders. Venlafaxine (Effexor®) is a "combination" antidepressant that has primarily SSRI-like effects in low doses and TCA-like effects (without cardiac problems) in higher doses. Effexor® and Effexor XR® have some positive benefits in ADHD treatment. Buproprion (Wellbutrin SR®, Zyban®) has serotonin and dopamine activity and is moderately to highly effective in ADHD treatment. It is a good choice for adolescents, adults, or clients with substance-abuse problems. Side effects of antidepressant medications are generally low, with sedation and tremors prominent in TCAs, and insomnia or GI upset with SSRIs. Chapter 8 discusses these medications more in-depth.

OPPOSITIONAL DEFIANT DISORDER

Oppositional defiant disorder occurs in up to half of all children with ADHD. It is charac-

terized by a recurrent pattern of negative, defiant and hostile behavior toward authority figures (and sometimes peers) to a degree that is not developmentally appropriate. The *DSM-IV-TR* criteria for oppositional defiant disorder are as follows:

1. A pattern of negative, hostile and defiant behavior lasting at least 6 months with four or more of the following:

    a. often loses temper

    b. often argues with adults

    c. often defies adults or refuses to comply with requests or rules

    d. often deliberately annoys people

    e. often blames others for his or her mistakes or poor behavior

    f. often touchy or easily annoyed by others

    g. often angry and resentful

    h. often spiteful or vindictive

Like all psychiatric disorders, the symptoms must be at a level that is detrimental to the child and interferes with functioning (social or family relationships, academic achievement). The behaviors seen cannot be attributed to another psychiatric disorder such as major depression or a psychotic disorder.

Oppositional defiant disorder children are unpleasant to live with. They seem to be frequently argumentative and defiant. Parents describe them as stubborn, resistant to redirection, inflexible, or argumentative. Testing limits is common as is verbal aggression and a refusal to take responsibility for one's actions. It is important to note, however, that this disorder is also a disorder of deficit and the child may not be at all happy with the behaviors. Low self-esteem and depression can occur easily in children with an oppositional defiant disorder, and they always seem to be in conflict with others. Oppositional defiant disorder symptoms usually begin before age 8, initially in the home setting. The symptoms will later generalize to other places such as school. Oppositional defiant disorder is more common in families with at least one member that has a history of major depression, and in families with significant conflict or marital discord.

Treatment for oppositional defiant disorder consists of individual and family therapy focusing on the dynamics in the family and ways to structure the environment so that the child is not dominating all family interactions. Behavior modification techniques are also useful. Medications are not particularly helpful, although an underlying depressive disorder should be carefully considered. Antidepressants may be of some benefit.

CONDUCT DISORDER

The main features of a conduct disorder are repetitive and persistent patterns of behavior in which the rights of others or social rules are consistently violated. Diagnostic criteria for conduct disorder include the following:

1. A persistent pattern of behavior in which the rights of others, or major societal norms or rules, are violated. At least three of the following must be seen over the previous 12 months (with at least one in the past 6 months):

Aggression to people and animals

   a. bullies, threatens, or intimidates others

   b. initiates physical fights

   c. has used a weapon that can cause physical harm

   d. has been physically cruel to people

   e. has been physically cruel to animals

   f. has stolen while confronting a victim (e.g., mugging)

   g. has forced someone into sexual activity

Destruction of property

   h. has engaged in fire-setting with the intent of causing damage

   i. has deliberately destroyed others' property

Deceitfulness or theft

   j. has broken into someone else's house, building or car

   k. often lies or "cons" others

   l. has stolen items of nontrivial value (e.g., shoplifting)

Serious violation of rules

   m. stays out at night regardless of parental curfew (before age 13)

   n. has run away from home overnight at least twice (or once if a lengthy period of time)

   o. often truant from school (beginning before age 13)

Conduct disorders are specified as mild, moderate, and severe depending on the number of problems and degree of harm to others. Children or adolescents with this disorder often act aggressively toward others and they display little empathy or concern for the feelings of others. They may feel justified in their behaviors, as they may perceive others as having hostile intentions (a paranoid disorder should be ruled out when diagnosing conduct disorder). Feelings of guilt or remorse are often absent. Poor frustration tolerance, recklessness, irritability, and temper outbursts are associated features as are promiscuity, gang activity, and drug use. Suicide ideation and attempts occur at a higher than average rate.

Children with conduct disorder are more likely to have parents with antisocial personalities, and to be raised in homes that are harsh, abusive, or lack supervision. In certain environmental situations, some behaviors consistent with conduct disorder may be socially adaptive (inner-city high-crime areas, war-ravaged countries), and the diagnosis should only be made when the behavior is indicative of an underlying dysfunction within the client. Children with conduct disorder are at risk of developing other psychiatric disorders, or of displaying adult criminal behaviors.

Treatment for conduct disorder almost invariably involves the court system. Court-ordered counseling may have some impact on future behaviors. Psychiatric assessment should be done to rule-out any other mental health disorders that may be responsive to medication intervention. Children and adolescents with severe conduct disorders often have one or more residential placements in mental health or juvenile detention facilities.

CHRONIC MOTOR OR VOCAL TIC DISORDER

Motor tics are sudden, rapid and recurrent motor movements that occur involuntarily several times a day, nearly every day, throughout a period of more than 1 year. Vocal tics are explosive vocalizations, also involuntary, that must occur nearly every day for more than a year. Both motor and vocal tics have an onset prior to age 18, and the direct effects of a medication, drug, or neurological disorder may not cause them. Transient tics (motor or vocal tics lasting less than 1 year) occur in children at a rate as high as 20% (Coffey, Biederman, Geller, Spencer, Park, Shapiro, & Garfield, 2000). Multiple motor and vocal tics lasting greater than 1 year is known as Tourette's disorder.

TOURETTE'S DISORDER

Tourette's disorder (TD) is a neuropsychiatric condition that occurs in approximately 4 per every 10,000 children in the United States (Coffey et al, 2000). It is higher in boys than in girls, and the onset is usually around age 6-7. The disorder may be life long, or it may spontaneously remit. The severity, frequency, disruptiveness and variability of the tics can wax and wane over time, and the characteristics of the tics can change without warning. Common simple motor symptoms

include eye blinking, facial scrunching, or grimacing, neck jerking, head turning, tongue protrusion, or licking. Complex tics may involve stooping, walking, twirling, or other multi-step activities. Vocal tics may be expressed as grunts, squeaks, squeals, sniffs, snorts, coughs, barks, throat clearing, or whole words or phrases. Coprolalia is a complex vocal tic involving the uttering of obscenities that is present in less than 10% of individuals with Tourette's disorder (*DSM-IV-TR*). Chronic tic symptoms can be extremely embarrassing to the client and lead to fears of rejection or humiliation in social situations.

Tourette's disorder has been associated with a number of other psychiatric problems (Table 14-3), in particular anxiety disorders (50%), ADHD (50-75%), and OCD (25%). Children with Tourette's disorder often present a complicated clinical picture.

TABLE 14-3: CO-OCCURRENCE OF TOURETTE'S DISORDER WITH OTHER PSYCHIATRIC DISORDERS

Disorder	% co-occurrence
Any psychiatric disorder	94%
Attention-deficit/hyperactivity	50-75%
Obsessive-compulsive disorder	25%
Other anxiety disorders	50%
Major depression	49%
Oppositional defiant disorder	58%
Bipolar disorder	14%
Speech and language disorder	24%
Enuresis	33%
(Coffey et al., 2000)	

The causes of Tourette's disorder are unclear. Genetic studies are underway and several neurotransmitters have been implicated. Dopamine receptor hypersensitivity has been the primary hypothesis for tic disorder and Tourette's disorder (Coffey, 2002).

Therapy is not indicated for the specific treatment of tic disorders or Tourette's disorder; however, counseling is extremely useful for the comorbid conditions, especially when self-esteem problems and depression occur. Mild cases may benefit from education, support, and monitoring alone.

MEDICATION INTERVENTIONS FOR TIC DISORDERS

Pharmacotherapy is essential for tics that have a significant impact on functioning or that cause emotional distress. First line treatment recommendations are the alpha-adrenergic medications Tenex® and Catapres®; if either of these medications is ineffective or poorly tolerated, then new-generation antipsychotics are the most effective treatment, primarily Risperdal®, Abilify™, Zyprexa®, or Geodon®. Older antipsychotics such as haloperidol (Haldol®) and pimozide (Orap®) are highly effective but much greater in side effects. TCAs have been useful in tic disorders combined with ADHD. SSRIs help with Tic disorders, combined with depression or anxiety, but they have little direct action on the tics themselves. Anxiolytics such as clonazepam (Klonopin®) may be used for short-term treatment. The use of stimulants to treat ADHD is controversial as stimulants may precipitate tic symptoms. There is no clear evidence that stimulant-induced tics are particularly harmful to the client, thus the clinician must make a careful consideration of cost versus benefit.

DISRUPTIVE BEHAVIOR DISORDER CASE STUDY

Isaac is a 6½-year-old boy who is referred for an evaluation at the end of first grade for problems with hyperactivity and temper tantrums. His mother reports that he gets angry over something every day, sometimes several times a day, and starts screaming, throwing things, hitting, or kicking. He does not harm himself during these episodes. The examiner notes that Isaac is running up and down the halls while in the waiting room. In the office, he is talkative and loud but quite cheerful; he is interested and curious about his surroundings; he plays with Legos® for a few minutes, trucks for a few minutes, then scribbles a picture, and announces he is ready to leave. He scatters the toys around the office without putting anything away. He also tries to play with the office computer and phone, and open the desk drawers. He even grabs an apple off of the desk and starts to eat it. Isaac's mother reports that his grades are very poor and he will have to attend summer school in order to be advanced to second grade. His citizenship grades are also poor with comments about out-of-seat behaviors, pushing or touching others, and interrupting her frequently. During the session, the examiner also notices "animal sounds" (squeaking, grunting, and throat clearing) of which the child seems unaware. Every few minutes, Isaac rolls his head back and rapidly blinks, then scrunches up his nose and sniffs. The mother states he has been doing this since he was 4 years old. The medical history reveals a normal prenatal period with a full-term delivery weight of 9 lb, 11 oz. Isaac was a healthy neonate who was rarely ill, but was very active as a toddler and frequently sustained bumps and bruises from climbing too high or riding his bike too fast. There are no allergies or current medications. He is sleeping fine at present. His language development has been normal, but some mild phonological problems persist and he is receiving speech therapy at school. Toilet training has been problematic — he is dry all day but wets the bed nearly every night and his mother puts him in Pull-ups® to sleep. He is of average weight and height for his age. A social history reveals an intact family with both biological parents and five children. Isaac is the youngest of four boys and one girl (ages range from 7-17). His father is a full-time mechanical engineer, his mother works part-time in *a daycare center. There is a family history of mild depression on the mother's side, and one older sibling has been diagnosed with ADHD. Isaac has few same-age friends, and spends most of his time at home playing with his 9-year-old brother. They are mutually very aggressive with one another.*

The examiner determines the following diagnoses:

Attention-deficit/hyperactivity disorder — combined type

Tourette's disorder

Phonological disorder

Enuresis, primarily nocturnal

Parent education is completed regarding the diagnosis and medication options, and the child is prescribed Concerta® 18 mg at 7 a.m., with Risperdal® .25 mg twice a day (b.i.d.) at 7 a.m. and 4 p.m., and Imipramine 10 mg at bedtime (h.s.).

NURSING CARE PLAN

Problem Listing

- Bed-wetting
- Problems with social skills
- Hyperactivity
- Risk for harm due to impulsivity
- Speech problems
- Aggressive acting-out
- School failure
- Short-attention span
- Chaotic home life
- Potential for low self-esteem
- Low frustration tolerance
- Poor academic performance

Priority Nursing Diagnosis

Poor frustration tolerance and self-control related to inability to control self as evidenced by daily tantrums and aggressive acting-out.

Long-term Goal

Client will demonstrate improved self-control and a reduction in tantrums.

Short-term Objectives

1. Client will stop hitting others.
2. Client's temper tantrums will be reduced from daily to 1-2 per month.
3. Parents will report better management and prevention of temper outbursts.

Nursing Interventions

1. Assist the parents in making a list of triggers that precipitate tantrums.
2. Discuss ways in which precipitants can be reduced or eliminated (e.g., not taking the child into the store if he usually has tantrums there).
3. Educate the parents as to effective use of time-outs.
4. Educate the client as to the use of personal time-outs.
5. Help the client learn to recognize signs of increasing tension and frustration.
6. Demonstrate and ask the parents to practice safe, therapeutic holds that may be necessary to prevent harm to others during tantrums.
7. Discuss the importance of providing support and reassurance to the client after a tantrum occurs, while discussing how things could have been handled differently.
8. Help the parents to identify ways to restructure the home environment in order to increase a sense of predictability and routines.

EXAM QUESTIONS

CHAPTER 14
Questions 93-100

93. A child with ADHD

    a. listens well and tries hard to please adults.

    b. completes assigned schoolwork with minimal supervision.

    c. does not listen well or follow through on assigned tasks.

    d. is usually put into special education classes at school.

94. Children with ADHD have poor academic performance because of

    a. problems with lower than normal IQ testing.

    b. problems with teachers who don't know how to manage the disorder.

    c. poor concentration and attention-span, and distractibility.

    d. parents who don't supervise or assist with homework.

95. ADHD management consists of the three core interventions of

    a. medications, school conferences, and physical exams.

    b. individual therapy, group therapy, and school conferences.

    c. family counseling and individualized educational plans.

    d. parent education, behavior management training, and medications.

96. A medication that is frequently prescribed for ADHD treatment is

    a. Haldol®.

    b. Paxil®.

    c. Concerta®.

    d. Aricept®.

97. Side effects to stimulant medications may include

    a. a loss of appetite, insomnia, and tic development.

    b. an increased appetite along with improved sleep patterns.

    c. decreased concentration and attention span.

    d. pacing, tremors, and other signs of extrapyramidal syndrome.

98. A child with oppositional defiant disorder will demonstrate a pattern of

    a. hyperactive and impulsive behaviors.

    b. negative, hostile, and defiant behaviors.

    c. disorganized and confused behaviors.

    d. criminal behaviors such as stealing.

99. An adolescent who bullies, intimidates others, lies, and steals probably has a(n)

    a. oppositional defiant disorder.

    b. attention-deficit/hyperactivity disorder.

    c. conduct disorder.

    d. early onset psychotic disorder.

100. Motor tics as seen in Tourette's disorder are defined as

    a. writhing worm-like movements with a gradual onset.

    b. sudden, rapid, and recurrent muscle movements.

    c. jerking movements with tremors and poor muscle control.

    d. a sudden loss of muscle tone and weakness.

This concludes the final examination. An answer key will be sent with your certificate so that you can determine which of your answers were correct and incorrect.

APPENDIX A

CULTURE-BOUND SYNDROMES

(*Diagnostic and Statistical Manual of Mental Disorders*, 4th ed., *Text Revision*. (2000). American Psychiatric Association, pp. 844-849.)

amok: "A dissociative episode characterized by a period of brooding followed by an outburst of violent, aggressive, or homicidal behavior directed at people and objects." The syndrome is described as primarily prevalent in males. Symptoms may include "persecutory ideas, automatism, amnesia, exhaustion, and a return to premorbid state."
Malaysia, Laos, Philippines, Polynesia (cafard or cathard), *Papua New Guinea, and Puerto Rico* (mal de pelea), *and among the Navajo* (iich'aa)

ataque de nervios: "Commonly reported symptoms include uncontrollable shouting, attacks of crying, trembling, heat in the chest rising into the head, and verbal or physical aggression. Dissociative experiences, seizurelike or fainting episodes, and suicidal gestures are prominent in some attacks but absent in other. A general feature...is a sense of being out of control." Attacks frequently occur in response to a stressful event.
Latinos for the Caribbean, Latin Americans, Latin Mediterraneans

bilis and **colera** (also called **muina**): "Symptoms can include acute nervous tension, headache, trembling, screaming, stomach disturbances, and, in more severe cases, loss of consciousness. Chronic fatigue may result from the acute episode. The underlying cause...is thought to be strongly experienced anger or rage. The major effect is to disturb core body balances."
Latino populations

boufee delirante: "A sudden outburst of agitated and aggressive behavior, marked confusion, and psychomotor excitement...sometimes accompanied by visual and auditory hallucinations or paranoid ideation."
West Africa, Haiti

brain fag: "A condition experienced by high school or university students in response to the challenges of schooling...somatic symptoms are usually centered around the head and neck and include pain, pressure or tightness, blurring of vision, heat, or burning."
West Africa

dhat: "Severe anxiety and hypochondriacal concerns associated with the discharge of semen, whitish discoloration of the urine, and feelings of weakness and exhaustion."
India, Similar to **jiryan** *(India),* **sukra prameha** *(Sri Lanka),* and **shen-k'uei** *(China)*

falling-out or **blacking-out:** "sudden collapse, which sometimes occurs without warning but sometimes is preceded by feelings of dizziness or "swimming" in the head...eyes are usually open but the person claims an inability to see. The person usually hears and understands what is occurring around him or her but feels powerless to move."
Southern United States, Caribbean groups

ghost sickness: "A preoccupation with death and the deceased…symptoms can be attributed to ghost sickness, including bad dreams, weakness, feelings of danger, loss of appetite, fainting, dizziness, fear, anxiety, hallucinations, loss of consciousness, confusion, feelings of futility, and a sense of suffocation."
American Indian Tribes

hwa-byung (wool-hwa-byung): "Anger syndrome" "Symptoms include insomnia, fatigue, panic, fear of impending death, dysphoric affect, indigestion, anorexia, dyspnea, palpitations, generalized aches and pains, and a feeling of a mass in the epigastrium."
Korea

koro: "An episode of sudden and intense anxiety that the penis (or, in females, the vulva and nipples) will recede into the body and possibly cause death" "Koro at times occurs in localized epidemic form in east Asian areas."
Malaysian origin, South and East Asia: Chinese (**shuk yang, shook yong, suo yang**); *Assam* (**jinjinia bemar**); *Thailand* (**rok-joo**)

latah: "Hypersensitivity to sudden fright, often with echopraxia, echolalia, command obedience, and dissociative or trancelike behavior. More frequent in middle-aged women."
Malaysian or Indonesian origin, Siberian groups (**amurakh, irkunii, ikota, olan,myriachit,** and **menkeiti**); *Thailand* (**bah tschi, bah-tsi, baah-ji**); *Ainu, Sakhalin, Japan* (**imu**); *Philippines* (**mali-mali, silok**).

locura: "A severe form of chronic psychosis… symptoms exhibited by persons with locura include incoherence, agitation, auditory and visual hallucinations, inability to follow rules of social interaction, unpredictability, and possible violence."
Term used by Latinos in the United States, Latin America

mal de ojo: "A Spanish phrase translated into English as "evil eye." Children are especially at risk. Symptoms include fitful sleep, crying without apparent cause, diarrhea, vomiting, and fever in a child or infant. Sometimes seen in adults (especially females)."
Mediterranean cultures and throughout the world

nervios: "Both a general state of vulnerability to stressful life experiences and to a syndrome brought on by difficult life circumstances. Common symptoms include headaches and "brain aches," irritability, stomach disturbances, sleep difficulties, nervousness, easy tearfulness, inability to concentrate, trembling, tingling sensations, and **mareos** (dizziness with occasional vertigo-like exacerbations)."
Common idiom of distress in Latin America and Latinos in the United States, Greeks in North America (**nevra**)

pibloktoq: "An abrupt dissociative episode accompanied by extreme excitement of up to 30 minutes' duration and frequently followed by convulsive seizures and coma lasting up to 12 hours." "During the attack the individual may tear off his or her clothing, break furniture, shout obscenities, eat feces, flee from protective shelters, or perform other irrational or dangerous acts."
Arctic and Subarctic Eskimo communities

qi-gong psychotic reaction: "An acute, time-limited episode characterized by dissociative, paranoid, or other psychotic or nonpsychotic symptoms that may occur after participation in the Chinese folk health-enhancing practice of qigong."
Chinese

rootwork: "a set of cultural interpretations that ascribe illness to hexing, witchcraft, sorcery, or the evil influence of another person. Symptoms may included generalized anxiety and gastrointestinal complaints (e.g., nausea, vomiting, diarrhea), weakness, dizziness, the fear of being poisoned, and sometimes fear of being killed (voodoo death)."

Southern United States in both African American and European American populations, Caribbean or Latino societies (**mal puesto, brujeria**)

running syndromes: "Conditions characterized by a sudden onset of a high level of activity, a trancelike state, potentially dangerous behavior in the form of running or fleeing, and ensuing exhaustion, sleep, and amnesia for the episode."

Native Peoples of the Arctic (**pibloktoq**), *Miskito of Honduras and Nicaragua* (**grisi siknis**)*, Navajo "frenzy" witchcraft, Western pacific Cultures* (**amok**)

sangue dormido: "sleeping blood" "Pain, numbness, tremor, paralysis, convulsions, stroke, blindness, heart attack, infection, and miscarriage."

Portuguese Cape Verde Islanders and their immigrants

Shenjing shuairuo: "A condition characterized by physical and mental fatigue, dizziness, headaches, other pains, concentration difficulties, sleep disturbance, and memory loss. Other symptoms include gastrointestinal problems, sexual dysfunctions, irritability, excitability, and various signs suggesting disturbance of the autonomic nervous system."

Chinese

shen-k'uei, shenkui: "A label describing marked anxiety or panic symptoms with accompanying somatic complaints for which no physical cause can be demonstrated. Symptoms include dizziness, backache, fatigability, general weakness, insomnia, frequent dreams and complaints of sexual dysfunction. Symptoms are attributed to excessive semen loss."

Taiwan, China

shin-byung: "Anxiety and somatic complaints (general weakness, dizziness, fear, anorexia, insomnia, gastrointestinal problems), with subsequent dissociation and possession by ancestral spirits."

Korean

spell: "A trance state in which individuals "communicate" with deceased relative or with spirits. At times....associated with brief periods of personality change."

African Americans, European Americans

susto "fright" or "soul loss", a.k.a. **espanto, pasmo, tripa ida, perdida del alma, chibih:** "an illness attributed to a frightening event that causes the soul to leave the body and results in unhappiness and sickness. Symptoms may appear any time from days to years after the fright is experienced. It is believed that in extreme cases, susto may result in death. Typical symptoms include appetite disturbances, inadequate or excessive sleep, troubled sleep or dreams, feeling of sadness, lack of motivation to do anything, and feelings of low self-worth or dirtiness. Somatic symptoms include muscle aches and pains, headache, stomachache, and diarrhea. Ritual healings are focused on calling the soul back to the body and cleansing the person to restore bodily and spiritual balance."

Latinos in the United States, Mexico, Central America, South America

taijin kyofusho: "This syndrome refers to an individual's intense fear that his or her body, its parts or its functions, displease, embarrass, or are offensive to other people in appearance, odor, facial expressions, or movements."
Japan

zar: "A term applied to the experience of spirits possessing an individual. Persons possessed by a spirit may experience dissociative episodes that may include shouting, laughing, hitting the head against a wall, singing, or weeping. Individuals may show apathy and withdrawal, refusing to eat or carry out daily tasks, or may develop a long-term relationship with the possessing spirit. Such behavior is not considered pathological locally."
Ethiopia, Somalia, Egypt, Sudan, Iran, other North African and Middle Eastern societies

APPENDIX B

NURSING ASSESSMENT AND DATA BASE (ADULT)

Client's Name: _____ Date: _____ MRN #: _____

Legal Status: ( ) Voluntary ( ) Involuntary: ( ) 24 hr immediate detention: Begins: _____

Ends: _____

( ) 72 hr emergency detention: Begins: _____

Ends: _____

( ) Temporary or Regular Commitment

Date of Birth: _____

Reason for Admission:

Previous Psychiatric Treatment:
Where?   When?

Medical Assessment:

BP: _____ HR: _____ RR: _____ Temp: _____ Ht: _____ Wt: _____

Allergies:

Medical History:

Integumentary:
Musculoskeletal:
Cardiac:
Respiratory: Cigarettes? _____ How many? _____
Gastric:
Urological:
Neurological:
Other:

Surgery History:

Alcohol or Drug Use:
What?   Last Used?

Current signs of alcohol/drug withdrawal?

Current Medications:

185

NURSING ASSESSMENT AND DATA BASE (pg.2)
ADULT

Client's Name: _____**Date:** _____ MRN #: _____

Review of Systems:

Sleep problems?

Nutritional concerns?

Acute or chronic pain?

Medication side effects?

Reproductive issues?

Other physical health issues:

Psychosocial History:

With whom does client live? _____

Identified significant other: _____ Phone: _____
             Release of Info signed? ( ) Yes ( ) No: reason _____

Children? ( ) Live with client: Ages? _____
             ( ) Live elsewhere: With whom? _____

Employment status: ( ) Employed: Where? _____
                   ( ) Unemployed: Chief source of income_____
                   ( ) Disabled: Type of disability _____
School status: ( ) High school, GED or higher education
                   ( ) Less than high school education: Learning disabilities? _____
                   ( ) Currently in school: Where? _____

Health Care Insurance coverage? Type: _____
             Does this policy cover prescription medications? ( ) Yes ( ) No ( ) Don't know

Support Systems:

Who does client identify as chief source of support? _____
Religious affiliation? ( ) Yes   Type: _____
                ( ) No

Mental Status Assessment:

Overall Appearance:

Behavior:

Mood and Affect:

NURSING ASSESSMENT AND DATA BASE (pg.3)
ADULT

Client's Name: _____Date: _____ MRN #: _____

Thought Processes and Organization:

Thought Contents:

    Primary focus of thoughts:

    Any hallucinations or delusions?

    Any suicidal thoughts/urges?

        Plan:

    Any homicidal thoughts/urges?

        Directed toward:

        Duty to warn? ( ) No ( ) Yes Whom:_____

    Memory impairments:

    Concentration problems:

Insight into illness:

Judgment:

Strengths: (Attributes that will assist client in recovery.)

Problem Listing: (Identify problems the client is experiencing.)

_____   _____
Nurse's Signature   Date

APPENDIX C

CASE STUDIES AND SAMPLE NURSING CARE PLANS
Case Studies as seen in Chapters 4-14

SCHIZOPHRENIA CASE STUDY

Jim is a 46-year-old man diagnosed with schizophrenia, paranoid type. He first became ill at age 19 when he came home from his freshman year of college to tell his parents that CIA agents had attempted to make contact with him using the computer lab in his dormitory. He has been hospitalized six times since, with one state hospitalization lasting 18 months after he assaulted his therapist (he accused the therapist of planting listening devices in his apartment). Jim has been put on the decanoate injectable form of the antipsychotic haloperidol (Haldol®), which he receives once a month at the mental health center. The nurse notes that Jim is rocking back and forth, rubbing his fingertips together, blinking rapidly, and smacking his lips. He is also taking the anticholinergic medication benztropine (Cogentin®) to control his tremors.

He weighs 278 lb at a height of 5'11". His blood pressure is 168/110 with a heart rate of 96 and a respiratory rate of 24. Jim tells the nurse that he drinks two pots of coffee a day, and smokes two to three packs of cigarettes. He is complaining about difficulty going to sleep before 4:00 a.m. — then he is unable to waken until 1:00 p.m. the following day. Jim also reports ongoing auditory hallucinations that are derogatory in nature. The "voices" tell him, "You are worthless. They're coming to get you! They'll lock you up again! Watch out!"

NURSING CARE PLAN

Problem Listing

- Poor nutrition — overweight
- Elevated blood pressure
- Shortness of breath
- Sleep cycle disturbance
- Caffeine abuse/dependence
- Nicotine dependence
- Auditory hallucinations
- Probable tardive dyskinesia
- Threats to self-esteem due to derogatory hallucinations

Nursing Diagnoses

1. Imbalanced nutrition: more than body requirements related to excessive intake of food as evidenced by weight of 278 lb at 5'11".

2. Ineffective health maintenance related to knowledge deficit as evidenced by blood pressure reading of 168/110.

3. Sleep pattern disorder related to excess intake of caffeine late at night as evidenced by a pattern of sleeping 4:00 a.m.-1:00 p.m.

4. Disturbed sensory perceptions: auditory hallucinations related to disease process as evidenced by patient report of "hearing voices."

5. Impaired physical mobility related to antipsychotic medication treatment as evidenced by symptoms of tardive dyskinesia.

Long-term Goal

Client will have improved physical and mental health status with a decreased risk for cardiac or respiratory disease.

Short-term Objectives

1. Client will reach a goal weight of 200 lbs by the end of 6 months.

2. Client will demonstrate BP readings consistently less than 140/90.

3. Client will go to sleep by 11:00 p.m. nightly.

4. Client will report decreased or eliminated auditory hallucinations.

5. Client will decrease caffeine and nicotine use by 50% in 6 months.

6. Client will verbalize the importance of regular physical activity in improving mobility.

Nursing Interventions

1. a. Educate the client about the importance of good nutrition for health.

   b. Facilitate a dietitian consult.

   c. Assist the client in identifying ways to build activity into the daily routine.

   d. Weigh the client weekly to monthly to assess progress.

2. a. Check BP with each monthly injection.

   b. Facilitate a medical exam with a family care provider to determine if an antihypertensive agent is needed.

3. a. Educate the client about the relationship between caffeine and insomnia.

   b. Teach the client relaxation techniques to utilize at bedtime.

   c. Encourage the client to set alarm clock for 8:00 a.m. daily and to get up.

   d. Advise the client to not take naps.

   e. Teach the client that cigarettes will keep him awake (not to smoke after 10:00 p.m.).

4. a. Discuss using as needed (p.r.n.) medications with the client.

   b. Educate the client about techniques to distract from the hallucinations (such as listening to music).

5. a. Assist the client in setting up a schedule to decrease caffeine and nicotine use.

   b. Suggest that the client use half-caffeinated and half-decaffeinated coffee.

6. a. Assist the client in incorporating activity into a daily schedule and teach gentle stretching techniques.

DEMENTIA CASE STUDY

Chip is a 72-year-old man who is living with his adult daughter and her family. His family physician suspected dementia when Chip began having difficulty in finding his way home from the grocery store. A neurology consult and MRI scan provided further evidence to support the disorder, and the neurologist prescribed Aricept® 10 mg a day. Most of the time, Chip is oriented to his surroundings and pleasant and cooperative with his family. He has been having increasing problems in the evening with confusion and recently became quite agitated and left the house at 11:00 p.m. "to go to work." Chip is a retired telephone lineman. After one of these episodes, his family physician prescribed 100 mg of amitriptyline (Elavil®) at bedtime in an attempt to help him sleep better. Three nights after taking this medication, Chip became extremely agitated and was yelling out, "Get them out of here! Get those men away from those lines before they blow!" His family had to call an ambulance to get him transported to the emergency department where he was sedated and then admitted to the medical-psychiatric unit. His admitting diagnoses were substance-induced delirium, and dementia of the Alzheimer's type. Elavil® was dis-

continued and in 2 days he was able to return home to his family.

NURSING CARE PLAN

Problem Listing

- Potential for injury
- Fear
- Family support needed

Nursing Diagnoses

1. Risk for injury related to drug toxicity as evidenced by acute delirium and agitation.
2. Fear secondary to a belief in threat or harm as evidenced by delusional statements.
3. Caregiver role strain related to increasing illness of client as evidenced by progressive dementia and attempts to leave the house.

Long-term Goal

Both client and family will receive the level of support needed to ensure ongoing positive relationships while maintaining a high standard of safety.

Short-term Objectives

1. Client will not sustain injury during period of delirium.
2. Client will demonstrate reduced fear by displaying a calmer demeanor and following simple directions.
3. Family will report an increased level of satisfaction with community resource awareness and availability by the time client is ready for discharge.

Nursing Interventions

1. Staff will monitor client closely and administer medications p.r.n.
2. Staff will assess for the need of temporary, soft wrist restraints during the acute phase of the agitation and delirium.
3. Staff will administer fluids and maintain a patent IV line.
4. Staff will use a soft, comforting voice tone and inform client of his safety during all procedures.
5. Staff will allow family members to remain at bedside as desired during hospitalization period.
6. Staff will provide social service resources and information on local caregiver support programs to family prior to client's anticipated discharge date.

ALCOHOL DEPENDENCE CASE STUDY

Maggie is a 38-year-old woman who has been employed as a real estate agent for the past 10 years. She graduated high school and completed 4 years of a business degree before landing this lucrative position for a large company. In high school, Maggie drank some with her friends. She had her first blackout at her senior prom — later she found out that she was dancing on the tables and making a fool of herself. In college, she attended various fraternity parties and had another blackout episode. This time she awoke to find herself naked and in bed with two men. She had no memory of the preceding events. Maggie continued to drink socially on weekends, and then she started taking prospective customers out during the week. Soon she found herself having wine with lunch, a cocktail or two after work, then several more in the evening at home. After Maggie's mother suddenly died of an aneurysm, her drinking escalated further to the point that she started to call in sick to work or go home early. She got her first DUI arrest while driving back to the office after showing a house. Her second DUI arrest (while at work) 2 months later cost her both her job and her driver's license. Unemployed, her drinking started to spiral out of control and she was always either intoxicated or sick. One night, Maggie started to vomit blood in copious amounts. Frightened, she called 911 and was rushed to the emergency department where she had to repair a ruptured esophageal varicoele. She was detoxified after 5 days, and started attending AA meetings while in the hospital. Maggie learned that she was an alcoholic, and would always be an alcoholic. She agreed to see a therapist and continue to attend AA meetings once discharged. Maggie relapsed three more times before she was able to reach 2 years of sobriety and become a sponsor for another woman.

NURSING CARE PLAN

Problem Listing

- GI bleeding
- Poor nutrition
- Ineffective coping
- Insomnia
- Alcohol withdrawal: tremors, dizziness, diaphoresis, elevated BP and heart rate
- Anxiety

Priority Nursing Diagnosis

Potential for harm due to alcohol withdrawal as evidenced by tremors, elevated vital signs, anxiety, diaphoresis, and dizziness.

Long-term Goal

Client will be safely detoxified in a medically supervised setting.

Short-term Objectives

1. Client will have a consistent BP reading of less than 130/90.

2. Client will have a heart rate reading of less than 100.

3. Client will report less anxiety and fewer tremors.

4. Client will not develop hallucinations or other signs of psychosis.

Nursing Interventions

1. Assess BP, heart rate and respirations every 2 hours and p.r.n.

2. Administer ordered benzodiazepines liberally every 2 hours and p.r.n.

3. Administer antiemetics as needed.

4. Encourage sipping of electrolyte replenishing fluids continuously.

5. Monitor intake and output.

6. Assess for blood in emesis or in stools.

7. Provide a bland, light diet for the first 48-72 hours of detoxification (unless NPO).

8. Keep environment quiet and nonstressful by turning down lights, keeping temperature at a comfortable level, and keeping noise to a minimum.

9. Restrict visitors if necessary.

10. Provide emotional support to client and family.

11. Once first few days of detoxification are complete, educate client as to processes of alcohol addiction (tolerance, dependence, withdrawal).

12. Make referrals to appropriate agencies including AA meetings.

SUBSTANCE DEPENDENCE CASE STUDY

Simon is a 40-year-old man with a long history of back problems. He was employed as a bricklayer/hodcarrier for 20 years, and injured his back through repeated heavy lifting on the job. The resultant back spasms caused him to be bedridden for days to weeks at a time. In an effort to obtain relief, Simon's family physician placed him on muscle relaxants (Flexeril®) four times a day and gave him hydrocodone 5mg/acetaminophen 500 mg (Lortab® 5/500) tablets to take as needed. Simon had some initial pain relief, but soon found that the Lortab® "stopped working." He increased his dose to every 4 hours, and then he started to take 2 tablets at a time. He quickly ran out and his physician refused to prescribe more, but offered him a referral to a pain management clinic. Feeling somewhat desperate, Simon called his dentist to report chronic pain secondary to an infected tooth. The dentist called in a prescription for Percocet® until Simon could be seen. After getting the prescription, Simon cancelled the dental appointment. By now he was taking up to 30 tablets of painkiller a day — some were his wife's "old" prescriptions and some were purchased from friends. Simon also scheduled and kept appointments with four different doctors to have his back pain evaluation. All of them gave him pain pills — some with 2 or 3 refills. When Simon was near to running out, he would go to the local emergency department (ED) and invariably would receive a Demerol® injection and a prescription. This pattern of behavior continued despite family concerns until Simon began vomiting and turned sallow in color. He was again taken to the ED, but this time his diagnosis was acute hepatitis secondary to acetaminophen overdosage. In the emergency room, Simon was given Narcan® and had an nasogastric-tube placed for a stomach lavage. He was then hospitalized and placed on Mucomyst® every 4 hours around the clock for 3-days with BID acetaminophen levels and daily liver enzymes. Simon reported feeling "like I've been hit by a Mack truck." He was tremulous and diaphoretic. He alternated between chills and flushing. He experienced nausea, vomiting, diarrhea, muscle cramps, and back spasms so intense that he was in tears much of the first 2 days. After he became more medically stable, the physician prescribed Neurontin® for the chronic pain and gave him some ibuprofen for generalized discomfort and trazodone (Desyrel®) to aid in sleep. On

discharge, a referral was made (and kept) to a pain clinic where Simon received physical therapy combined with steroid injections, topical analgesics (Lidocaine® patches), heat, massage, and education regarding the importance of activity and weight loss.

NURSING CARE PLAN

Problem Listing

- Chronic pain
- Inadequate coping responses to deal with pain
- Drug-seeking behaviors
- Opioid withdrawal symptoms
- Potential for injury
- Insomnia

Priority Nursing Diagnosis

Ineffective coping with chronic pain as evidenced by drug-seeking behaviors and opioid addiction.

Long-term Goal

Client will have minimal to no back pain without the use of addictive substances.

Short-term Objectives

1. Client will attend physical therapy appointments and practice exercises at home.

2. Client will verbalize an understanding of the dangers of overuse of prescribed medications.

3. Client will report a decrease in pain to a level that does not interfere with the enjoyment of life and daily activities.

Nursing Interventions

1. Educate the client and his family as to the processes of addiction (tolerance, dependency, withdrawal).

2. Discuss with the client alternative pain management techniques that may be useful including heat, massage, gentle exercise, and stretching.

3. Facilitate education into alternate medication options.

4. Help the client to identify learned behaviors in response to pain.

5. Explain to the client that 100% remission is not the goal and help the client to identify what level of pain may be tolerable.

6. Assist the client in scoring or rating pain on a scale of 1-10 so that the client can better communicate how it feels to health care providers (and self).

7. Assist the client in identifying and listing diversional activities to use at home.

8. Teach the client relaxation techniques (breathing techniques) to be utilized when pain level is increasing.

DEPRESSION CASE STUDY

*D*ebra *is a 54-year-old woman with no significant mental health history. She recently saw her family physician for vague complaints of fatigue, restlessness, and insomnia, which she felt were attributed to "going through the change." Debra's menstrual cycles became irregular then ceased entirely 1 year ago. Her physician recommended light exercise and a hormone replacement medication. One week later, Debra's husband noted that she no longer had any desire to go with him to flea markets (a favorite weekend activity) and she seemed listless and apathetic. Her sleep problems worsened and she found herself waking at 2:00-3:00 a.m. and unable to return to sleep. Her appetite started to decrease and she frequently "forgot" to make the family's evening meal as she usually did complaining of exhaustion. Debra started experiencing intense headaches nearly every day causing her to always keep the curtains drawn and the lights low. Her symptoms exacerbated rapidly following the death of her favorite cat due to old age. She began crying uncontrollably,*

even at supermarkets, and refused to go out in public anymore. Her husband noticed that she was in the house either pacing in an agitated, purposeless manner or she was staring off into space; even television could no longer distract her. Over the course of a month, she lost 15 lb from her 145-lb frame. She started to talk to her husband about "the hereafter" and what to do with her possessions "once I am gone." He insisted she see a therapist who immediately referred Debra for an evaluation with a psychiatric Clinical Nurse Specialist. The CNS took a thorough history to rule out any concomitant illnesses or drug/alcohol abuse, and ordered some baseline lab tests including a thyroid panel. The lab tests showed only a mild dehydration, but were otherwise normal. The CNS then prescribed Lexapro® (escitalopram) 10 mg once daily for depression plus a p.r.n. of Restoril® (temazepam) 15 mg h.s. for the insomnia. The therapist continued to work with Debra and her husband educating them both as to the illness of depression. He also helped Debra to learn some cognitive strategies to deal with day-to-day stressors. Debra reported an improved mood and sleep within a week. By the fourth week her husband stated she was "nearly back to herself." At the end of 6 weeks, Debra felt "normal" again and was able to terminate therapy, but agreed to continue taking the antidepressant. She no longer needed the p.r.n. sleeping medication.

NURSING CARE PLAN

Problem Listing

- Fatigue

- Changes in ADLs

- Insomnia

- Hopelessness

- Dysmenorrhea

- Suicidal thoughts

- Weight loss
- Altered family relationships
- Crying episodes
- Poor concentration
- Impaired decision-making
- Socially isolating self

Priority Nursing Diagnosis

Self-care deficit related to persistent depressed mood as evidenced by fatigue, hopelessness, poor hygiene, and social isolation.

Long-term Goal

Client will return to her previous functioning level.

Short-term Objectives

1. Client will not remain in bed all day.

2. Client will resume previous activities with husband (e.g., flea markets) within 2 weeks.

3. Client will resume household responsibilities (e.g., cooking meals) within 2 weeks.

Nursing Interventions

1. Assist the client in making a daily living schedule and post this in a prominent place in the home.

2. Help the client and husband to identify places to go for diversional recreation no less than twice a week.

3. Provide medication education to the client and husband.

4. Assist the client in evaluating sleep patterns and develop a sleep hygiene plan (e.g., reduced caffeine, getting up at the same time every day, h.s. sedatives) to facilitate improved sleeping patterns.

5. Instruct the client to engage in 20-30 minutes of brisk walking daily (preferably outdoors if the weather is permitting).

6. Instruct the client in a healthy diet with plenty of fruits and vegetables. Daily multivitamins can be recommended.

7. Encourage the client to continue her regular church attendance.

BIPOLAR I DISORDER CASE STUDY

Pablo is a 22-year-old man who has completed 2 years of fine arts study in a major university. Always creative, he started to find himself unable to stop painting or sketching until well into the night. Eventually, he found himself able to stay up for more than 48 hours with little effort. His friends commented that he always seemed to be "on a natural high" and he was "fun to be around." Pablo was very productive in his painting, but he started to miss classes as he began to think that there was nothing they could teach him that he didn't already know. After a few weeks, Pablo's irregular hours and poor eating habits caused him to look thin and tired. His energy level became more frenetic and agitated, and his friends stopped visiting — now he seemed to be irritable and short-tempered, plus they were tired of hearing about his "genius talent." One day, when Pablo had been awake for 4 consecutive days, he called his parents to tell them about the "great opportunity" he would have if they would buy him a plane ticket to Paris. He was certain that the Louvre' would hang his paintings and give him a private showing on the spot, after all he felt he was "channeling the spirit and soul of Van Gogh." When his parents questioned this, Pablo became agitated saying he would get the money "somehow" and no one would stop him. Subsequently, Pablo was arrested for attempted robbery of a convenience store. The arresting officer put in his report that "the perpetrator was shouting obscenities and appeared to be talking to some he kept calling 'Vince.'" Pablo was admitted to a secure psychiatric facility on an immediate detention order. He initially required four-way restraints and chemical sedation. He was started on Depakote ER® (valproic acid) and titrated to 2,500 mg/day. Additionally, he was prescribed Zyprexa® at 20 mg h.s. and was given p.r.n. doses of Ativan® (lorazepam). After 7 days inpatient, he was discharged to his parents' home for further recuperation.

NURSING CARE PLAN

Problem Listing

- Altered mood states — agitation, excitability
- Altered thoughts — delusions of grandeur, ideas of reference, auditory hallucinations
- Inadequate sleep
- Poor nutrition
- Knowledge deficit regarding his illness or medications
- Potential for harm to self or others

Priority Nursing Diagnosis

Potential for harm to self or others related to altered thoughts (grandiosity, ideas of reference) as evidenced by extreme agitation and irrational behaviors.

Long-term Goal

Client will no longer demonstrate any evidence of psychosis.

Short-term Objectives

1. Client will not harm self during the hospital stay.
2. Client will not harm others (staff, visitors) during the hospital stay.
3. Client will demonstrate compliance with recommended medication treatment.

Nursing Interventions

1. Nurse will administer p.r.n. medications at the first sign of increasing agitation.
2. Nurse will educate the client in relaxation techniques to help in reducing anxiety.

3. Seclusion and restraints will be utilized by staff in a judicious manner and only when absolutely necessary.
4. Staff will adapt a nonconfrontational, supportive approach with client to minimize potential misperceptions due to altered thoughts.
5. Staff will keep the client in a private room until all risk for assaultive behavior has passed.
6. Staff may elect to restrict visitors if client's behavior is inappropriate.

GENERALIZED ANXIETY DISORDER CASE STUDY

Casey is a 16-year-old girl who is being seen in the pediatrician's office for complaints of stomachaches nearly every day at school. She has been going to the nurse's office frequently and asking the health aid to call her mother. Occasionally she will also request an acetaminophen tablet for headaches. Casey was an honor roll student her freshman year, but this year her grades have dropped to a B-C average. During her appointment, she tells the nurse that she is worried that she won't be able to get into college with such poor grades. A college student was recently abducted while out riding her bicycle in Casey's hometown; she was later found murdered. Casey has been asking her mother to carry a cellular phone when she goes out jogging in the evenings, and she calls her every 15 minutes. When her mother doesn't return promptly in 45 minutes, Casey calls her cellular phone in a panic. One time she called 911 to report her mother as missing when the cell phone batteries went dead. At home, Casey has reported trouble falling asleep at night before 1:00 a.m., and then she has vague nightmares of being chased by vampires and zombies from "The Night of the Living Dead." She feels tired during the day at school. Casey's parents divorced 14 years previously, but she has a stable home life at both her mother and her father's homes. Lately she hasn't wanted to go out with friends or leave home very often, unless her mother leaves with her (even then she really wants to remain at home). Medically, Casey is healthy. She has no allergies or history of any medical problems. She does not take any medications. She was a full-term infant and met all of her developmental milestones on target. There is a positive history of anxiety and depression on her mothers' side of the family, but none presently. The pediatrician diagnoses Casey with gastritis secondary to a generalized anxiety disorder. After consulting with the parents, she prescribes Zoloft® 50 mg once-daily plus Zantac® 150 mg at bedtime (h.s.).

NURSING CARE PLAN

Problem Listing

- Stomachaches
- Headaches
- Nonspecific worries
- Social isolation
- Feelings of being unsafe
- Sleep disturbance
- Feelings that her family is unsafe

Priority Nursing Diagnosis

Anxiety related to perceived threats to integrity of self and family as evidenced by persistent worries, stomachaches, and a drop in academic performance.

Long-term Goal

Client will have anxiety reduced to a level that no longer interferes with her functioning.

Short-term Objectives

1. Client will report no stomachaches.
2. Client will stop calling mother every 15 minutes while mother is jogging.

3. Client will bring grades back to the previous A-B average.

Nursing Interventions

1. Establish a sense of rapport and trust with the client by utilizing the active listening techniques of open-ended questions, clarifying, validating, and reflecting feelings.
2. Remain nonjudgmental and noncritical of the client.
3. Teach the client relaxation breathing to be utilized in times of stress. Practice these techniques until client has mastered them.
4. Talk the client through a guided imagery session and how to utilize guided imagery when alone.
5. Consult with parents regarding client's need for reassurance and support.
6. Provide medication education for SSRIs.
7. Assist the client in developing a plan for completing homework in a timely manner.
8. Ask the client to keep a daily journal of thoughts and feelings, and how they impacted behavior for that day.
9. Encourage client to resume social activities with peers.

ANOREXIA NERVOSA CASE STUDY

Brittany is an attractive, petite cheerleader in the 8th grade. She wants to make the high school squad next year, but some of her friends tell her that the competition is really hard and you have to be perfect to get selected. Brittany goes through a growth spurt the summer before high school and she grows to 5'7" and puts on 10 lb, bringing her weight up to 135 lb. One of the boys from her school sees her at the Mall, and says, "Hey, you been eating all summer or what?" Brittany becomes determined to lose weight. She starts to skip breakfast, then lunch. Soon she is eating once a day. She tells her family that she is going to be a vegetarian "because meat is gross." She starts exercising 2-3 hours every evening. Her weight starts to come off and she starts to get compliments from her friends. At 120 lb her mother suggests that she looks a little thin, but Brittany only sees fat around her thighs and stomach. Soon she is only eating a little lettuce (no dressing) and an apple for the day. Her weight continues to drop, and she notices some of her hair falling out in the shower. Although she is still exercising, she stops going out with friends because she is too tired. At 105 lb her menstrual cycles cease. By now, her parents are very concerned and they take her to a pediatrician. He tells them it's "just a phase, a lot of girls go through," so they try not to worry. By Christmas, Brittany weighs only 90 lb and she looks emaciated. She tells her best friend, Jennie, that she "just needs to lose a little more." At 84 lb Brittany faints at school and is rushed to the hospital. She is admitted to the intensive care unit for premature ventricular contractions and starvation syndrome. A psychiatric referral is made as well. Once stabilized, she is referred to an eating disorder specialist who meets with her and her family once a week to help Brittany develop some understanding of the disorder, and set a reasonable goal weight for maintenance.

NURSING CARE PLAN

Problem Listing

- Calorie intake less than body requirements
- Cardiac arrhythmia
- Amenorrhea
- Distorted body perception
- Low self-esteem

Priority Nursing Diagnosis

Alteration in nutrition, less than body requirements, related to self-induced eating disorder, as evidenced by a body weight of 84 lb with a height of 5' 7".

Long-term Goal

Client will return to a body weight of 115 lb or above.

Short-term Objectives

1. Client will gain 1-2 pounds every week.
2. Client will eat a combination of carbohydrates, fats and proteins.
3. Client will identify three positive qualities about self not related to physical appearance or weight.
4. Client will verbalize an understanding of her diet plan.

Nursing Interventions

1. Daily calorie count — instruct family and client for home usage.
2. Monitor fluid intake and electrolyte balances.
3. Educate the client about healthy food choices.
4. Provide support and encouragement with rewards for healthy weight gain.
5. Refer client to appropriate therapy (individual and group) and support services in the community.

SOMATIZATION DISORDER CASE STUDY

*B*ertha is a 45-year-old divorced woman who has been going to doctors since she was 22 years old. Her ex-husband was abusive and an alcoholic. She suffers from chronic fatigue, headaches, diarrhea (or sometimes constipation), and funny tingling feelings in her legs, hot flashes, and dizziness. At age 25 she had a total abdominal hysterectomy for irregular cycles. Persistent abdominal pain resulted in an exploratory laparoscopy at *age 27. Bertha also had a cholecystectomy and incidental appendectomy for small gallstones when she was age 32. When her surgical wound became infected and separated, she had to have a mesh placed. At home, she "takes to her bed" frequently with migraine headaches. Her three adolescent children are left to feed and care for themselves, with very little supervision. Bertha "threw out her back" carrying groceries one day last year, and she takes prescription pain medications several times a day. Most of her family won't visit anymore — they have grown tired of hearing her persistent complaining and tales of medical treatments gone awry. The rheumatologist put Bertha on nonsteroidal anti-inflammatory medications for her joint pain, the surgeon gave her antacids for her "heartburn," and her family doctor gives her hormone replacement plus sleeping pills (for her chronic insomnia). Bertha is increasingly depressed and doesn't understand why no one can tell her what is wrong with her. Her 16-year-old son came home from school to find her unconscious with empty pain pill bottles. She was rushed to the hospital and admitted to the intensive care unit.*

NURSING CARE PLAN

Problem Listing

- Chronic pain — headaches, backaches, abdominal pain, joint pain
- Gastrointestinal symptoms — diarrhea, constipation, heartburn
- Sexual symptoms — hot flashes, surgically-induced menopause
- Neurological symptoms — weakness, numbness, and tingling extremities
- Psychological symptoms — depression, suicide attempt, low self-esteem
- Social problems — family rejection, no diversional activities, unemployed, children grown and more independent

Priority Nursing Diagnosis

Chronic low self-esteem related to long-standing reliance on others to meet her emotional needs as evidenced by the development of numerous physical ailments that require frequent medical evaluation.

Long-term Goal

Client will develop supportive relationships in the community to meet her needs for support and reassurance.

Short-term Objectives

1. Client will identify two activities that she can do on a weekly basis (may include volunteer work).
2. Client will be able to list at least three positive attributes.
3. Client will be able to have a 30-minute conversation with another adult and not discuss any physical complaints.
4. Client will report improved relationships the three children.

Nursing Interventions

1. Assist the client in identifying community resources and volunteer opportunities.
2. Support the client in finding and listing three positive attributes.
3. Gently the redirect client away from physical complaints during conversations and toward social or life events.
4. Provide a nonjudgmental, caring approach.
5. Refer for family therapy for client and children.

BORDERLINE PERSONALITY DISORDER CASE STUDY

*D*anny *is a 32-year-old man with a history of over 10 psychiatric hospitalizations for superficial cuts to his wrists, overdoses, or suicidal threats. He has also been in jail twice: once for a DUI charge, and once for domestic violence. Danny has been in the hospital four times in the past 6 months alone. One year ago, Danny's third wife left him after only 18 months of marriage and filed a restraining order to prevent him from contacting her. Upon examination, Danny tells the nurse that, "life isn't worth living unless you have someone to love you." He also states that "I don't know what I'll do if you make me leave the hospital again." Danny goes on to report that the staff on the previous shift "wouldn't listen to me" and that one of the technicians had threatened to "beat me up if I didn't straighten up and quit lying." Danny feels that the social worker is the only one who really understands him. Since the divorce, Danny has been homeless and staying in shelters. He isn't working "because my ex-wife screwed that up for me" and he has no insurance or source of income. He states his family abused him as a child and, "I won't have anything to do with them." The nurse finds that he has a history of unstable relationships, some of them heterosexual and some of them with same-sex partners. Danny also tends to downplay his substance abuse history stating, "It's really not a problem. I just drink when I'm depressed." Danny's primary admission diagnosis is Adjustment disorder with depressed mood, but he is also diagnosed with a borderline personality disorder.*

NURSING CARE PLAN

Problem Listing

- Potential for harm to self or to others

- Poor coping strategies to deal with life stressors

- Lack of housing, income, other resources

- Impaired social interactions

Priority Nursing Diagnosis

Potential for harm to self related to impulsivity as evidenced by a history of previous attempts when under severe psychosocial stress.

Long-term Goal

Client will identify and utilize more effective means of dealing with stressors other than harming himself.

Short-term Objectives

1. Client will verbally and in writing contract with staff not to harm himself during the hospital stay.

2. Client will verbalize self-harm urges to staff prior to acting on them.

Nursing Interventions

1. Staff will perform 15-minute safety checks to assess clients' well-being.

2. Staff will assist the client in listing five activities to perform to prevent harming himself (for example, journaling, exercising, or calling support hotlines).

3. Staff will assist the client in identifying both precipitants to self-harm behaviors as well as thought processes (cognitive interpretations) of events that led up to those feelings.

DEVELOPMENTAL DISORDER CASE STUDY

*M*atthew *is an 8-year-old boy with autistic disorder who presents in the health care facility for an increase in aggressive behaviors. His mother reports that he was first recognized as autistic at age 3. He has difficulty relating to others, and* *prefers to play alone with his toy cars (stacking them and twirling their wheels), which he can do for hours. Lately, he has started to lick the backs of his hands repetitively and they are red and chapped. Whenever family members or school-teachers ask him to stop playing or licking and attend to tasks-at-hand (such as schoolwork or a family meal), he starts to yell and rock back and forth. If he is touched, he strikes out violently against anyone he can reach. Matthew has difficul-ty in using language to express his needs, and at times he doesn't seem to understand what is being asked of him. In addition to the autism diagnosis, academic testing has revealed an IQ of 72. Medical findings are as follows: 4'10", 75 lb, BP 110/58, heart rate 110; hands are chapped and reddened; nails are bitten to the quick; nocturnal enuresis 4-5 nights out of 7; rare diurnal enuresis; rare enco-presis; sleep is decreased with an onset of 11 p.m. and awake by 5 a.m. daily; appetite is erratic; increased motor activity and impulsive striking out.*

Matthew is placed on Luvox® 25 mg at bedtime to be titrated to 50 mg at bedtime (h.s.) in 1 week and DDAVP nasal spray bilateral nares at bedtime (h.s.). A toileting routine was also discussed with his parents to facilitate in his staying dry at night.

NURSING CARE PLAN

Problem Listing

- Bedwetting 4 or 5 nights out of 7
- Sleep onset problems
- Red, chapped hands (potential for infection)
- Impulsive, aggressive behaviors
- Inflexibility with changes in routines

Priority Nursing Diagnosis

Risk for violence directed toward others related to poor impulse control as evidenced by strik-ing out at caregivers when redirected.

Long-term Goal

Client will learn alternative ways to communi-cate his needs without resorting to aggression.

Short-term Objectives

1. Client will not strike out more than once a month.

2. Client will demonstrate "personal time-outs" when feeling upset prior to striking out.

Nursing Interventions

1. Educate parents to recognize the four stages of crisis escalation:

   a. Trigger (events that precipitate acting-out)

   b. Escalation (behaviors that indicate increas-ing tension)

   c. Acting-out (striking out or destructive behaviors)

   d. De-escalation (calming down).

2. Educate parents as to means of dealing with each stage as it occurs:

   a. Trigger — identify precipitants then work to reduce or eliminate them.

   b. Escalation — recognize signs of tension (e.g., pacing or rocking), then help child to redirect his energy or to take a personal time-out.

   c. Acting-out — place child in safe time-out area. May use as needed medications if they are available.

   d. De-escalation — talk with child about what led to time-out (e.g., "In this family we don't hit other people," reassure child, for example, "You're a good boy and we love you.")

3. Ask parents to log acting-out behaviors for one week, then help them to analyze the triggers, how they responded to signs of escalation and acting-out, and how the process of de-escala-tion occurred.

4. Educate parents in ways to help their child transition between activities in order to reduce stress-responses (e.g., giving 5-minute warnings, getting eye contact prior to giving directions, and asking him to repeat directions.)

DISRUPTIVE BEHAVIOR DISORDER CASE STUDY

Isaac is a 6 ½-year-old boy who is referred for an evaluation at the end of first grade for problems with hyperactivity and temper tantrums. His mother reports that he gets angry over something every day, sometimes several times a day, and starts screaming, throwing things, hitting, or kicking. He does not harm himself during these episodes. The examiner notes that Isaac is running up and down the halls while in the waiting room. In the office, he is talkative and loud but quite cheerful; he is interested and curious about his surroundings; he plays with Legos® for a few minutes, trucks for a few minutes, then scribbles a picture, and announces he is ready to leave. He scatters the toys around the office without putting anything away. He also tries to play with the office computer and phone, and open the desk drawers. He even grabs an apple off of the desk and starts to eat it. Isaac's mother reports that his grades are very poor and he will have to attend summer school in order to be advanced to second grade. His citizenship grades are also poor with comments about out-of-seat behaviors, pushing or touching others, and interrupting her frequently. During the session, the examiner also notices "animal sounds" (squeaking, grunting, and throat clearing) of which the child seems unaware. Every few minutes, Isaac rolls his head back and rapidly blinks, then scrunches up his nose and sniffs. The mother states he has been doing this since he was 4 years old. The medical history reveals a normal prenatal period with a full-term delivery weight of 9 lb, 11 oz. Isaac was a health neonate who was rarely ill,

but was very active as a toddler and frequently sustained bumps and bruises from climbing too high or riding his bike too fast. There are no allergies or current medications. He is sleeping fine at present. His language development has been normal, but some mild phonological problems persist and he is receiving speech therapy at school. Toilet training has been problematic — he is dry all day but wets the bed nearly every night and his mother puts him in Pull-ups® to sleep. He is of average weight and height for his age. A social history reveals an intact family with both biological parents and five children. Isaac is the youngest of four boys and one girl (ages range from 7-17). His father is a full-time mechanical engineer, his mother works part-time in a daycare center. There is a family history of mild depression on the mother's side, and one older sibling has been diagnosed with ADHD. Isaac has few same-age friends, and spends most of his time at home playing with his 9-year-old brother. They are mutually very aggressive with one another.

The examiner determines the following diagnoses:

Attention-deficit/hyperactivity disorder — combined type

Tourette's disorder

Phonological disorder

Enuresis, primarily nocturnal

Parent education is completed regarding the diagnosis and medication options, and the child is prescribed Concerta® 18 mg at 7 a.m., with Risperdal® .25 mg twice a day (b.i.d.) at 7 a.m. and 4 p.m., and Imipramine 10 mg at bedtime (h.s.).

NURSING CARE PLAN

Problem Listing

- Bed-wetting
- Problems with social skills
- Hyperactivity

- Risk for harm due to impulsivity
- Speech problems
- Aggressive acting-out
- School failure
- Short-attention span
- Chaotic home life
- Potential for low self-esteem
- Low frustration tolerance
- Poor academic performance

Priority Nursing Diagnosis

Poor frustration tolerance and self-control related to inability to control self as evidenced by daily tantrums and aggressive acting-out.

Long-term Goal

Client will demonstrate improved self-control and a reduction in tantrums.

Short-term objectives

1. Client will stop hitting others.
2. Client's temper tantrums will be reduced from daily to 1-2 per month.
3. Parents will report better management and prevention of temper outbursts.

NURSING INTERVENTIONS

1. Assist the parents in making a list of triggers that precipitate tantrums.
2. Discuss ways in which precipitants can be reduced or eliminated (e.g., not taking the child into the store if he usually has tantrums).
3. Educate the parents as to effective use of time-outs.
4. Educate the client as to the use of personal time-outs.
5. Help the client learn to recognize signs of increasing tension and frustration.
6. Demonstrate and ask the parents to practice safe, therapeutic holds that may be necessary to prevent harm to others during tantrums.
7. Discuss the importance of providing support and reassurance to the client after a tantrum occurs, while discussing how things could have been handled differently.
8. Help the parents to identify ways to restructure the home environment in order to increase a sense of predictability and routines.

GLOSSARY

accommodation: Used by Piaget, accommodation refers to learning new information based on previous experiences. For example, a child learns that dogs are animals then he accommodates to include cats, horses, and cows as also being animals.

acting-out: A term used in mental health care to describe any aggressive or self-injurious behavior committed by another, usually in response to increasing levels of anxiety or tension but may also be a result of hallucinations or delusions.

affective flattening: Used to describe emotions, affective flattening refers to a blunting of emotional expression often seen in the disorder of schizophrenia.

agnosia: Refers to inability to recognize familiar objects, usually as a result of brain injury or dementia.

agoraphobia: A pathological fear of being in public places. Can vary in intensity from mild (unable to be in large crowds) to extreme (unwilling to leave the house).

agranulocytosis: A serious and sometimes fatal illness characterized by a significant reduction in white blood cells. Can be caused by illnesses or medications.

alogia (poverty-of-speech): A paucity of speech content that reflects a lack of abstraction in thoughts. Clients with this problem often respond minimally to questions and are unable to elaborate or provide details or embellishments.

amenorrhea: An absence of menstrual cycles. May be associated with normal changes related to menopause, or may be induced by disorders such as anorexia nervosa or medications.

amnesia: A defect in memory; an inability to recall parts or wholes of certain events or situations.

anorexia: A loss of appetite. May refer to self-restricting behaviors (anorexia nervosa) or may be caused by medical conditions (cancer treatment) or psychiatric disorders (depression).

anticholinergic: Usually used to refer to a medication action, anticholinergic drugs block nerve transmission through parasympathetic pathways resulting in reduced activity of the gastrointestinal and urinary tract, and reduced secretions, such as saliva or tears.

aphasia: Partial or total loss of the ability to speak, usually as a result of brain injury.

apraxia: An impaired ability to carry out purposeful movements, usually as a result of brain injury.

assimilation: A term used by Piaget to indicate how children learn; refers to learning new information by comparing it to previously learned data. For example, a child learns that a fly is an insect, and then assimilates to include ants, beetles, and wasps as insects as well.

ataxia: Staggering gait. Unsteadiness. Commonly seen in acute alcohol, sedative, or opioid intoxication. Also seen in other toxic reactions (heavy metal poisoning, and lithium toxicity).

avolition: An inability to initiate actions seen in individuals with neurological disorders (e.g., Parkinson's disease) or in schizophrenia. A tendency to have little motivation or activity level.

battered woman syndrome: A phenomenon of emotional exhaustion experienced by women who are in a domestic violence situation from which they feel they are unable to escape. Depression, hopelessness, helplessness, and suicidal thoughts may occur. Depersonalization experiences are common. Victim may become delusional or homicidal.

beneficience: The act of being kind or doing good.

blood dyscrasias: Refers to any abnormal condition of the blood.

bradykinesia: An abnormal slowing of motor movements as seen in disorders such as Parkinson's disease. Related to medical disorders, severe psychiatric disturbances, or older antipsychotic medications.

catalepsy (waxy flexibility): A state of prolonged rigid posture usually encountered in catatonic schizophrenia. Others can move the extremities and the client will hold them statue-like until they are moved again.

cataplexy (sleep paralysis): A sudden and complete state of paralysis brought on by shock, or experienced during the phase of sleep encountered immediately prior to waking. Associated with rapid eye movement (REM) sleep stages.

catatonia: A state of stupor and muscular rigidity encountered in the catatonic subtype of schizophrenia. The client does not move for long periods of time.

choreiform movements: Writhing, wormlike movements usually of the upper extremities or neck that are associated with tardive dyskinesia, but may also be caused by neurological disorders.

circumstantial thoughts: Thought patterns, reflected by speech, that do not get directly to the point but rather talk around the main topic for a period of time before eventually returning to finish the sentence or main idea.

cognitive: A general term that refers to mental acts such as reasoning, perception, intuition, and knowledge.

cognitive behavior therapy: A therapy model that teaches individuals to examine their preconceived ideas about events or situations, then examine how those ideas influence perceptions and interpretations, emotional responses and behaviors. The ultimate goal is to relearn how to interpret life events.

compulsions: An irrational urge to perform an action repeatedly, often without a logically reason to do so. Is often associated with obsessive thoughts.

concomitant: Occurring at the same time, or in conjunction with.

coprolalia: A rare form of vocal tic that is characterized by the expression, usually explosively, of socially unacceptable words or phrases such as curse words.

cross-tolerance: A phenomenon that is seen in substance-dependent clients where addictions to one substance can induce very high tolerance levels for similar substances. Most likely is related to elevated liver enzymes.

culture-bound syndromes: Psychologically driven behaviors or patterns of behavior that vary between cultures. May be representative of distinct disorders, but most likely they are a result of learned responses and differences in defining a psychiatric disturbance.

decompensate: A term used when a client with a psychiatric disorder is becoming symptomatic again after a period of relative stability.

defense mechanisms: Coping strategies utilized by clients in times of stress. First categorized and labeled by Sigmund Freud to explain behavioral reactions based on unconscious drives.

delirium tremens: Usually refers to alcohol withdrawal accompanied by vivid hallucinations, anxiety and tremors. Commonly referred to as "D.T.'s", delirium tremens often precede seizures.

delusions: Abnormal and false beliefs associated with a brain-based disorder. Can be expressed in a variety of ways (physical beliefs and paranoid beliefs) but all are real to the person experiencing them.

disinhibition: A loss of inhibitions usually caused by the effects of a substance (e.g., alcohol, drugs). Can also be associated with a brain injury or a disorder such as dementia. Disinhibited individuals will behave in ways in which they would normally be too embarrassed or reserved to do.

duty-to-warn: A legal term resulting from the 1976 case of Tarakoff v. The Regents of the University of California where the University was found negligent for not directly warning Ms. Tarakoff that her life had been threatened (thus denying her the opportunity to protect herself) when they had information revealed in a therapy session that she was going to be murdered. Mental health practitioners now each have an individual duty to warn others when there has been a threat made, even without the consent of the client.

dysmenorrhea: Irregular or abnormal menstrual cycles caused by medical illness or medication side effects.

dysphasia: A disorder of language caused by a learning disability or a brain lesion. May affect either expressive or receptive/expressive abilities to communicate.

dysphagia: A disorder of swallowing that may have medical or psychological causes.

dysphoria: A feeling of being ill at ease; commonly used in the mental health field to refer to an individual who looks sad or depressed.

dystonia: A neurological disorder that causes skeletal muscles to go into a spasm and contract. Psychiatrically, it is usually associated with the side effects of traditional antipsychotic medications. Dystonic reactions frequently involve the head, neck, trunk, or ocular muscles.

echolalia: A tendency to repeat words spoken by another. Usually seen in mental retardation or other developmental delays, brain injuries, and schizophrenia.

echopraxia: An involuntary repetition of the actions of others. Usually seen in mental retardation or other developmental delays, brain injuries, and schizophrenia.

encephalopathy: A general term that refers to any degenerative disease of the brain. Is often associated with chronic exposure to toxins including alcohol.

encopresis: The voluntary or involuntary passing of feces after age 4 in socially unacceptable places or at inappropriate times.

enuresis: The voluntary or involuntary passing of urine after age 5 in socially unacceptable places or at inappropriate times.

enzymes: Biological proteins that act as catalysts to trigger or accelerate chemical reactions.

erotomania: An abnormally strong sexual desire, or an obsession with another person accompanied by an unfounded belief that the other person returns those affections.

escalate: A term used in mental health care to indicate an increasing level of tension and anxiety by the client. Can be a precursor to acting-out.

euphoria: A feeling of exaggerated happiness or well-being often accompanied by increased activity. May be induced by drugs or associated with the mania phase of a bipolar disorder.

executive functioning: A term that refers to the brain's ability to dictate or rule, or organize the person's thoughts and behaviors. May be impaired from illnesses, injuries, or drugs.

extrapyramidal syndrome: Side effects of antipsychotic medications related to low dopamine levels in the extrapyramidal tract of the brain characterized by tremors, shuffling gait, stiff muscles, and a masklike facial expression.

failure to protect: A legal term used when a parent has knowledge that their dependent (child or adult) is endangered, but fails to act on the knowledge and allows the dependent to come to harm. Often used in child abuse and neglect cases.

fight-or-flight: A primitive physiological response to a perceived threat to the self characterized by increased adrenalin (epinephrine) levels, increased corticosteroids, a release of endogenous opiates, and other changes that prepare the organism to fight for protection or to run away.

flashbacks: A sudden reoccurrence of a memory or an experience that is unwanted by the individual; may be triggered by an event or situation similar to the original experience. Flashbacks occur in individuals with posttraumatic stress disorder, acute stress disorder, or following ingestion of a hallucinogenic agent.

flight-of-ideas: A description of thought processes that are unable to stay focused or on topic; one idea will cause the client to think of another idea and so forth until the individual loses track of the original thread of the conversation.

flooding: An experience where clients are suddenly exposed to an extreme anxiety provoking phenomenon from which they are unable to flee. May be part of a therapy plan in treating specific phobias or obsessive compulsive disorder.

folie á deux: Also called a shared delusional disorder, folie á deux refers to the adoption of the false beliefs of another usually based on a close relationship or proximity.

galactorrhea: The abnormal and excessive expression of breast milk. Galactorrhea is seen in nonpregnant clients in the psychiatric setting as a result of medications that elevate serum prolactin levels (traditional antipsychotics and risperidone).

general adaptation syndrome: A term coined by Hans Selye to describe the stages of adaptation to stress experienced by the human organism. Incorporates elements of Alarm, Resistance, and Exhaustion. Alarm is associated with fight-or-flight responses; resistance is associated with chronic anxiety and somatoform disorders; and exhaustion is associated with depression, dissociative disorders and posttraumatic stress.

grandiosity: A feeling that one has special abilities or traits that elevates one above the common man. May include a sense of entitlement or be demonstrated as arrogance.

grimacing: Scrunching up of the face as seen with pain. In the psychiatric setting this is usually recognized either as a symptom of schizophrenia, or as an indication of tardive dyskinesia associated with traditional antipsychotic medications.

guarded: Refers to a client who presents as evasive or paranoid, and is unwilling to share any personal information.

guided imagery: A form of relaxation therapy where a client is taught to imagine a calm, serene place and pretend that they are there.

habituation: The development of a tolerance for a substance that indicates the beginnings of a physiological addiction; a need for increasing amounts of the substance to accomplish the same effects.

hallucinations: The experience of false sensory perceptions: visual, auditory, olfactory, tactile, or gustatory.

holistic: Used in nursing and health care to mean the whole person: physical, emotional, and spiritual.

hypervigilance: A position of heightened alertness or awareness often accompanied by an exaggerated startle response and frequently seen in posttraumatic stress disorder or in paranoid delusions.

hypomania: A state of elevated moods and activity that represent a change from the baseline of the individual and that may be accompanied by impulsive behaviors or a decreased need for sleep. Does not require hospitalization and psychosis may not be present.

ideas of reference: A type of delusion where clients believe that mundane or irrelevant experiences in the world have a personal connection to them; such as the belief that the news reporter is secretly trying to send you a personal message regarding an impending terrorist attack. Also includes beliefs of telepathic abilities or thought insertion by others.

incest: Sexual abuse to a minor perpetrated by a family member.

insight: The act of developing awareness into the self that includes understanding one's own motivations, drives, impulses, and urges.

intellectual quotient: A standardized test usually referred to as "IQ" that measures the intellectual capability of a client and is used for educational planning. IQ tests have some cultural bias for non-English speaking persons.

intrusive thoughts: The experience of having unwanted thoughts come into the mind repeatedly and that usually require and inordinate amount of effort to overcome.

lacrimation: Fluid running from the tear ducts as seen in weeping, but without the emotional context of sadness.

lanugo: A fine, usually blond hair found on the bodies and faces of newborn babies that is lost within a few days to weeks. Lanugo can occur in clients with severe anorexia nervosa.

maladaptive: Coping mechanisms or behaviors employed by the client that do not help the client to cope adequately, and may be very detrimental. Examples include excess alcohol consumption, risk-taking behaviors, or self-mutilation.

maleficience: The act of wrongdoing or causing harm to another.

mania: The presence of an abnormally elevated, expansive, or irritable mood that is a clear change from baseline and that causes impairment in social relationships, or occupational or educational functioning. Clients with mania may sleep little and they may have psychotic symptoms or require hospitalization.

melatonin: A naturally occurring hormone that is produced by the body in response to daylight. Melatonin levels have an association to mood problems seen in seasonal affective disorder, and to jet lag.

mutism: The inability or refusal to speak in the absence of damage to the vocal cords or the brain. May be seen in children or adults who have been severely traumatized.

myopathy: Degenerative condition of the skeletal muscles causing problems with strength and stability. Can be related to neurological disorders, toxins, or infections.

negativism: A persistent and pronounced pessimistic outlook on life characterized by chronic disgruntlement.

neologisms: A phenomenon seen in schizophrenia and other brain-based disorders where an individual makes up words that are not in the standard dictionary.

neuroleptic malignant syndrome: A life-threatening syndrome where muscle tissue breaks down at an alarming rate and is accompanied by hyperthermia and elevated BP and heart rates. Causes of this syndrome are unknown, but it is thought to be associated with traditional antipsychotic mediations. Rates are higher in older adult women with other medical problems, or in clients taking both an antipsychotic and lithium.

neurons: Part of the physical makeup of the gray matter of the brain, a neuron is composed of a cell body with a large nucleus. Neurons transmit waves of electrical potential by using chemical elements called neurotransmitters.

neuropsychiatric: A term used to describe a disorder that has psychiatric or psychological expressions, but is associated with physical or neurological alterations.

neurosis: First used by Freud, a neurosis is a psychological disorder that does not alter the individual's perception of reality, primarily used for personality disorders and some anxiety disorders.

neurotransmitter: Neurotransmitters are the chemical messengers that move from one neuron to another and carry electrical action potential. The neurotransmitters most important in psychiatry are serotonin, dopamine, norepinephrine, acetylcholine, and gamma-aminobutyric acid.

obsession: A recurrent, unwanted thought that the individual can usually recognize as illogical or irrational (unless it occurs in children then there is less insight), but is unable to resist or prevent from occurring.

orientation: Used in nursing and health care to refer to an awareness of one's identity, surroundings, location, and time. Disorientation is seen in delirium and dementia disorders, and in acute substance intoxication.

PANDAS: An acronym that stands for Pediatric Autoimmune Neuropsychiatric Disorders Associated with Group A Beta-hemolytic Streptococci. PANDAS are usually sudden onset obsessive-compulsive or tic disorders that occur following a positive strep throat culture.

paradoxical reaction: An unexpected reaction to a medication that is opposite of the intended reaction. Often seen in children (e.g., an antihistamine causes agitation and hypomania), but benzodiazepines can cause paradoxical reactions in adult clients as well.

paranoia: A delusion that is characterized by an irrational belief that one is endangered, being followed, or being watched by others, or by governmental agencies.

pharmacodynamics: Refers to what a drug is designed to do, or the action of drugs on the physiology of the body (e.g., certain antidepressants block the reuptake of serotonin in the neurons).

pharmacokinetics: How a drug moves through the body. It involves absorption and distribution, metabolism, and excretion.

pica: The abnormal desire or compulsion to consume nonnutritive material (chalk, dirt, paint, or hair). May be associated with nutritional deficiencies, especially in pregnancy, or may have no known cause. More common in individuals with mental retardation or developmental delays.

piloerection: Commonly known as "goosebumps," an autonomic response to cold or fear that causes small muscles in the skin to contract and pull the hair upright. Also seen in opioid withdrawal.

polygenic polydipsia: A compulsive urge to drink fluids, particularly water, to a degree that overwhelms the body's ability to eliminate excess fluid via the kidneys resulting in dangerously low sodium and potassium levels through a dilutional effect. Thought to be related to the activities of certain medications on the thirst-control mechanisms in the brain, polydipsia can constitute a medical emergency.

poverty-of-speech (alogia): A paucity of speech content that reflects a lack of abstraction in thoughts. Clients with this problem often respond minimally to questions and are unable to elaborate or provide details or embellishments.

poverty-of-thoughts: An inability to think abstractly or to embellish or add details to thoughts.

priapism: A painful, unremitting erection associated with the medication trazodone. Although rare, it can constitute a medical emergency.

prions: A protein in the brain, the abnormal form of which is thought to be responsible for viral infections such as Creutzfeldt-Jakob syndrome (mad cow disease).

pseudodementia: A phenomenon where an individual with major depression presents with memory deficits similar to those seen in a dementia disorder. It is characterized by a fairly rapid onset, and an erratic and fluctuating course.

pseudoparkinsonism: Symptoms of Parkinson's disease that are caused by some medications, in particular antipsychotics, which have a nonspecific dopamine-blocking effect in the brain. The symptoms are reversed when the medication is withdrawn. Includes tremors, shuffling gait, stiff muscles, and a masklike facial expression.

psychoanalysis: The type of therapy first implemented by Freud and based on the premise that unconscious sexual tensions drive behaviors, and that change is accomplished by uncovering early childhood experiences.

psychomotor retardation: Severely slowed movements of the body accompanied by slowed or abnormal mental processes.

psychosis: A general term used in psychiatry to indicate a client who is suffering from hallucinations, delusions, or gross disorganization of thought processes. Psychosis is a descriptor and not a diagnosis.

relaxation training: A type of therapy commonly practiced by nurses that involves teaching the client to use a combination of deep breathing and muscle contractions and relaxations to achieve a calmer state. Often used in combination with guided imagery.

repression: The involuntary burying of memories into the subconscious usually related to a traumatic event or situation. The client is unaware of these memories unless there is a triggering stimulation associated with the original trauma.

restraint: The act of physically restricting the freedom of an client using manual, mechanical, or chemical means (forced medications). Designed to prevent harm to the client or to others. Would constitute assault and battery if not in a clinically supervised setting.

rhabdomyolysis: Breakdown of skeletal muscle usually associated with a neuroleptic malignant syndrome.

rhinorrhea: Excessive runny nose commonly seen in opioid withdrawal.

ruminative: An inability to stop thinking about something. Based on a cow chewing a cud, an individual may ruminate about finances, etc. May be associated with intrusive thoughts (thoughts that come unbidden), but differs from obsessions in that ruminations often have a real-life, rational basis.

saliorrhea: Excessive salivation often seen as a side effect to the antipsychotic clozapine.

seclusion: The restriction of a client's right to freedom by placing them in a locked or secure room. Constitutes illegal confinement if not done in a clinically supervised setting.

self-mutilation: The act of cutting, burning, or otherwise intentionally harming oneself, usually as a result of overwhelming emotional distress. Self-mutilation brings about a sense of relief and calm, which may be related to stimulation of endogenous opiates.

somatic: Of, or relating to the physical human body (as opposed to the mind). Somatic disorders are those that involve some perception of a physical symptom or problem.

speedball: The lethal combination of heroin and cocaine or amphetamine, snorted or injected, in order to get high. Cardiac arrest can result.

stereotypical behaviors: Rigid, fixed or nonproductive repetitive behaviors such as rocking, hand-flapping, or clapping that are often seen in developmental delays or mental retardation.

Stevens-Johnson syndrome: A painful, excoriating rash that can result as a side effect from some medications. Of concern in the mental health setting are the antiepileptics used for bipolar disorder (Lamictal®, Tegretol®).

stupor: A state of extreme mental dullness, cloudiness, or decreased consciousness where the individual can be aroused with a great deal of effort, but they have little awareness of their surroundings.

sundowning: A phenomenon that is seen in dementia disorders, particularly of the Alzheimer's type, where confusion and disorientation worsens as the evening progresses, and improves with daylight.

synesthesia: The experience while under the influence of an hallucinogenic agent that smells can be heard, sounds tasted, or music felt (a disorganization of sensory perceptions).

tangential: A thought process problem where thoughts branch off from one to another and the central theme or idea is lost.

tardive dyskinesia: A potentially irreversible side effect to antipsychotic medications (particularly the traditional ones) that is characterized by smooth and rhythmic muscular contractions of the head, neck or trunk, tongue thrusting, subvocalizations (such as grunting), or hand and finger movements.

teratogenic: Having to do with risk or harm to an unborn fetus. Teratogenic drugs are those that cause birth defects.

tic: A sudden and somewhat explosive motor or vocal spasm that occurs rapidly and without warning. Tics can exacerbate and remit spontaneously. They are more common in children, or they may be a side effect of stimulant medications.

time-out: A distinct period of time away from a triggering event or situation that allows the individual to regain a sense of self-control before returning to confront the situation.

torsades de pointes: A potentially lethal ventricular tachycardia in which electrical conduction in the heart follows an abnormal, circular pattern. Torsades de pointes can occur when depolarization of the heart muscle occurs during the critical part of repolarization, also referred to as the R-on-T phenomenon.

waxy flexibility (catalepsy): A state of prolonged rigid posture usually encountered in catatonic schizophrenia. Others can move the extremities and the client will hold them statue-like until they are moved again.

word salad: A disorder of thought processes where words within a sentence have no logical connection to one another, and the sentence does not make any sense. Seen in disorganized schizophrenia.

RESOURCES

American Academy of Child and Adolescent
  Psychiatry
www.aacap.org

American Nurses Credentialing Center
www.nursingworld.org/ancc

American Psychiatric Nurses Association
www.apna.org

American Psychological Association
www.apa.org

Centers for Disease Control and Prevention
  CDC Public Health Practice Program Office
  U.S. Department of Health and Human
  Services
www.phppo.cdc.gov

Children and Adults with Attention-
  Deficit/Hyperactivity Disorder (CHADD)
www.chadd.org

Center for the Study of Autism
www.autism.org

International Society of Psychiatric-Mental
  Health Nurses
www.ispn-psych.org

Markula Center for Applied Ethics
www.scu.edu/ethics

Minnesota Program Development, Inc.
  Domestic Abuse Intervention Project
www.duluth-model.org

National Alliance for the Mentally Ill (NAMI)
www.nami.org

National Council on Alcoholism and Drug
  Dependence
www.ncadd.org

National Institutes of Health (NIH)
www.nih.gov

National Institute for Occupational Safety and
  Health Administration (NIOSH)
www.cdc.gov

National Institute of Mental Health (NIMH)
http://www.nimh.nih.gov

National Institute on Alcohol Abuse and
  Alcoholism
www.niaaa.nih.gov

National Women's Health Information Center
www.4woman.gov

Surgeon General's Report on Mental Health
  and Minorities
www.mentalhealth.org

U.S. National Library and the National Institute
www.nlm.hih.gov

BIBLIOGRAPHY

Ackley, B.J., & Ladwig, G. B. (2002). *Nursing diagnosis handbook: A guide to planning care,* (5th ed.). St. Louis, MO: Mosby Year-Book.

Agronin, Marc E. (2002). The undertreated disease. *Eldercare, 2*(3), 8-10.

Alcoholics Anonymous. (1976). *The big book: The basic text for Alcoholics Anonymous* (3rd ed.). New York: Alcoholics Anonymous World Services, Inc.

American Academy of Child & Adolescent Psychiatry: National facts. (1999). *1999 Violence fact sheet.* Retrieved November 10, 2002, from: http://www.aacap.org/ingo_ families/NationalFacts/99ViolFctSh

American Psychiatric Association. (2000). *Diagnostic and Statistical Manual of Mental Disorders: Text Revision,* (4th ed.) Washington, DC: Author.

American Psychological Association: APA Ethics Office. (2002). *Ethics.* Retrieved January 4, 2003, from: http://www.apa.org/ethics

Bedard, L.R., & DeVolentine, J. (2000). Institutional case management applied to acute psychiatric care in correctional mental health. *Journal of Offender Rehabilitation, 30*(3-4), 21-34.

Center for Narcolepsy. (2003). *Fact Sheet.* Retrieved April 13, 2003, from: www.med.Stanford.edu

Coffey, Barbara. (2002). *Tics and Tourette's disorder.* Presented March 16, 2002, at the Conference on Child and Adolescent Psychopharmacology. March 15-17. Massachusetts General Hospital and Harvard Medical School, sponsors.

Coffey, B., Biederman, J., Geller, D., Spencer, T., Park, K., Shapiro, S., & Garfield, S. (2000). The course of Tourette's disorder: A literature review. *Harvard Review of Psychiatry, 8*(4), 192-197.

Coffey, B., Biederman, J., Smoller, J., Geller, D., Sarin, P., Schwartz, S., & Kim, G. (2000). Anxiety disorders and tic severity in juveniles with Tourette's disorder. *Journal of the American Academy of Child and Adolescent Psychiatry, 39*(5), 562-568.

DeBello, M., Schwiers, M.S., Rosenberg, H. L., & Strakowski, S.M. (2002). A double-blind, randomized, placebo-controlled study of quetiapine as adjunctive treatment for adolescent mania. *Journal of the American Academy of Child and Adolescent Psychiatry,* October, *41*(10), 1216-1223.

Dittmann, S., Forsthoff, A., Thoma, H., & Grunze, H. (2002). Clozapine as an add-on in the maintenance treatment of rapid cycling bipolar disorder. *Clinical Approaches in Bipolar Disorders, 1*(1), 31-33.

Domestic Abuse Intervention Project. (2003) Minnesota Program Development, Inc: National Training Project. Retrieved April 3, 2003, from: www.duluth-model.org

Fendrick, A.M., & Langa, K.M. (2002). The far-reaching effects of Alzheimer's disease. *Eldercare, 2*(4), 1-4.

Folstein, M.F., Folstein, S.E., & McHugh, P.R. (1975). Mini-Mental State. In L.S. Schneider, P.N. Tariot, & J.T. Olin (Eds.) (2000). *Manual of Rating Scales for the Assessment of Geriatric Mental Illnesses* (p. 19). Wilmington, DE: AstraZeneca Pharmaceuticals LP.

Fortinash, K.M., & Holoday Worret, P.A. (2003). *Psychiatric nursing care plans* (4th ed.). St. Louis, MO: Mosby, Inc.

Frye, M., Gitlin, M., & Altshuler, L. (2003). Foundational treatment: Treating acute mania. *Current Psychiatry,* (supplement).

Gabbard, G.O., & Lazar, S.G. (Eds.). (2002). Efficacy and cost effectiveness of psychotherapy. *American Psychiatric Association.* Retrieved November 17, 2002, from: http://www.psych.org/pract_of_psych/ispe_efficacy

Glick, R.L. (2002). Emergency management of depression and depression complicated by agitation or psychosis. In University of Rochester School of Medicine and Dentistry, *Psychiatric issues in emergency care settings,* (pp. 3-9).

Headlee, R., & Corey, B.W. (1948). *Psychiatry in nursing.* Binghamton, NY: Vail-Ballou Press, Inc.

Holman, A., & Cohen Silver, R. (2000). Primary care patients report high rates of trauma. In Today at UCI (Press Release). (2002, November 17). Retrieved November 17, 2002, from: http://www.today.uci.edu/news/release

Hughes, D. (2002, April). Sudden onset of obsessive compulsive disorder may point to PANDAS. *Neurology Reviews.com, 10*(4). Retrieved April 4, 2003, from: www.neurologyreviews.com

Keltner, N.L., Schwecke, L.H., & Bostrom, C.E. (2003). *Psychiatric nursing* (4th ed.). St. Louis, MO: Mosby, Inc.

Kern, M. (2003). Stages of change model. *Addiction Alternatives.* Retrieved July 6, 2003, from: www.aa2.org/philosophy/stagemodel

Kingsbury, S.J., Mohamed, F., Trufasiu, D., Zada, J., & Simpson, G.M. (2001, May). The apparent effects of ziprasidone on plasma lipids and glucose. *Journal of Clinical Psychiatry, 62*(5), 347-349.

Koller, E., & Doraiswamy, P.M. (2002). Olanzapine-associated diabetes mellitus. *Pharmacotherapy, 22*(7), 841-852.

Kruger, S., & Braunig, P. (2002). Clinical Issues in Bipolar Disorder during Pregnancy and the Postpartum Period. *Clinical Approaches in Bipolar Disorders,* (1), 65-71.

Manning, J.S. (2002, August). Beyond antidepressants: Bipolar spectrum illness presenting as complicated or refractory mood disorders in primary care. *Medscape Psychiatry and Mental Health: Clinical Update.* Available online: www.medscape.com

McGaha, A.C., & Stiles, P.G. (Eds.). (2001). *The Florida Mental Health Act (The Baker Act): 2000 Annual Report.* Louis de la Parte Florida Mental Health Institute: Department of Mental Health Law and Policy. Univ. of South Florida. Retrieved November 23, 2002, from: http://www.bakeract.fmhi.usf.edu

Markula Center for Applied Ethics. (2002). *The ethics connection.* Santa Clara University. Retrieved January 4, 2003, from: http://www.scu.edu/ethics

Mick, E. (2002). New understanding of ADHD as a chronic disorder. *Treating ADHD Across All Domains of Impairment,* (pp. 7-13). Sacramento, CA: Veritas Institute for Medical Education, Inc.

Nasrallah, H.A., & Smeltzer, D.J. (2002). *Contemporary diagnosis and management of the patient with schizophrenia.* Newtown, PA: Handbooks in Health Care, Co.

National Institute for Occupational Safety and Health (NIOSH). (1997). *Violence in the Workplace.* Retrieved April 4, 2003, from: www.cdc.gov/niosh

National Council on Alcoholism and Drug Dependence, Inc. (2001). Effects of prenatal exposure to a combination of illicit drugs, alcohol, or other drugs. *Nebraska Council to Prevent Alcohol and Drug Abuse Brochure.* Retrieved April 13, 2003, from: www.necoun cil.org

National Institute of Mental Health. (2001). *Mental disorders in America.* Department of Health and Human Services. Retrieved November 10, 2002, from: http://www.nimh.nih.gov/pulicat/ numbers

National Institute on Alcohol Abuse and Alcoholism. (2002). Alcohol and minorities: An Update. *Alcohol Alert (55).* U.S. Department of Health and Human Services. Retrieved January 4, 2003, from: http://www. niaaa.nih.gov

Nieves, M.R. (2003). Munchausen by Proxy Syndrome. *The Pediatric Bulletin, 5*(5). Retrieved April 20, 2003, from: www. home.coqui.net

Nulman, R., Rovet, J., Stewart, D., Wolpin, J., Pace-Asciak, P., Shuhaiber, S., et al. (2002). Child development following exposure to tricyclic antidepressants or fluoxetine throughout fetal life: A prospective, controlled study. *The American Journal of Psychiatry, 159*(11). Retrieved January 15, 2003, from: www. gateway2.ovid.com

Okasha, A., Arboleda-Flórez, J., & Sartorius, N. (Eds.). (2000). *Ethics, culture and psychiatry: International perspectives.* Washington, DC: American Psychiatric Press, Inc.

Perlis, R.H., Evins, A.E., Ogutha, J., & Sachs, G.S. (2002). Atypical antipsychotics in the treatment of bipolar disorder. *Clinical Approaches in Bipolar Disorder,* (1), 4-9.

Physicians' Desk Reference®. (57th ed.) (2003). Montvale, NJ: Thomson Healthcare.

Skidmore-Roth, L. (2003). *2003 Mosby's nursing drug reference.* St. Louis, MO: Mosby, Inc.

Spencer, T., Biederman, J., & Wilens, T. (2000, January). Pharmacotherapy of attention deficit hyperactivity disorder. *Psychopharmacology, 9*(1), 77-97.

Stein, Mark. (2002, December). Consequences of untreated and undertreated ADHD on social and adaptive functioning. *Treating ADHD Across All Domains of Impairment: A 3-part Series* (pp. 23-27). In J. Biederman, (Ed.) Sacramento, CA: Veritas Institutes for Medical Education, Inc.

Surgeon General's Report. (1999a). *Fact Sheet: African Americans.* Retrived January 4, 2003, from: http://www.mentalhealth.org

Surgeon General's Report. (1999b). *Fact Sheet: Asian Americans/Pacific Islanders.* Retrived January 4, 2003, from: http://www.mental-health.org

Surgeon General's Report. (1999c.). *Fact Sheet: Latinos/Hispanic Americans.* Retrived January 4, 2003, from: http://www.mentalhealth.org

Surgeon General's Report. (1999d). *Fact Sheet: Native American Indians.* Retrived January 4, 2003, from:http://www.mentalhealth.org

Surgeon General's Report. (1999e). *Chapter 2: The influence of culture and society on mental health, mental illness.* Retrived January 4, 2003, from:http://www.mentalhealth.org

The National Women's Health Information Center. (2003). *Women of color health data book: Factors affecting the health of women of color.* U.S. Dept. of Health and Human Services. Retrieved January 4, 2003, from: http://www.4woman.gov/owh/pub/woc/elderly

Treatment Advocacy Center. (2002). *Fact sheet: Historical view of mental illness crisis and debacle of deinstitutionalization.* Retrieved November 17, 2002, from: http://www.psych laws.org

U.S. National Library and the National Institute. (2001). *Medline Plus: Health information.* Retrieved November 23, 2002, from: http://www.nim.hih.gov/medlineplus/ency/articfle/001947

United States Census Bureau: Facts for features. (2001). *11th Anniversary of Americans with disabilities act (July 26).* Retrieved November 10, 2002, from:http://www.census.gov/Press-Release/www/2001

United States Constitution: 14th Amendment. Retrieved November 23, 2002, from: http://www.law.cornell.edu/constitution/constitution.amentdmentxiv

University of South Florida. *Transtheoretical Model/Stages of Change Overview.* Retrieved July 6, 2003, from: www.hsc.usf.edu

Whooley, M.A., & Simon, G.E. (2000). Managing depression in medical outpatients. *The New England Journal of Medicine, 343*(26), 1942-1950.

Wolraich, M. (1996). *Disorders of Development and Learning: A Practical Guide to Assessment and Management* 2nd ed. St. Louis, MO: Mosby, Inc.

INDEX

PRETEST KEY

Psychiatric Nursing: Current Trends in Diagnosis and Treatment

Question	Answer	Chapter
1.	b	1
2.	a	2
3.	d	2
4.	a	2
5.	b	3
6.	a	4
7.	c	5
8.	a	6
9.	d	7
10.	c	8
11.	a	8
12.	b	9
13.	d	9
14.	a	10
15.	b	11
16.	c	11
17.	d	12
18.	b	13
19.	a	14
20.	d	14

Western Schools® offers over 60 topics to suit all your interests – and requirements!

Clinical Conditions/Nursing Practice

Critical Care/ER/OR

Geriatrics

Hot Topics/Issues

Maternal-Child/Pediatrics/Women's Health

Professional Issues/Management/Law

Psychiatric/Mental Health

Visit us online at www.westernschools.com for these great courses – plus all the latest CE topics!

Online testing also available.

REV. 12/03